PCCN Review Book 2019 – 2020

PCCN Study Guide and Practice Test Questions for the Progressive Care Certified Nurse Exam

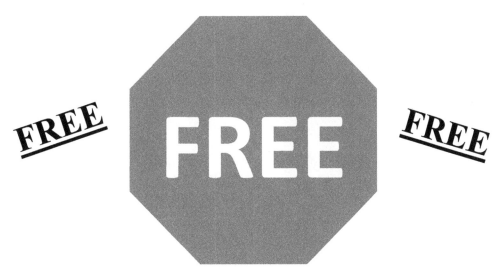

PCCN Essential Test Tips Video
from Trivium Test Prep!

Dear Customer,

Thank you for purchasing from Trivium Test Prep! We're honored to help you prepare for your PCCN exam.

To show our appreciation, we're offering a **FREE *PCCN Essential Test Tips* Video by Trivium Test Prep**. Our Video includes 35 test preparation strategies that will make you successful on the PCCN. All we ask is that you email us your feedback and describe your experience with our product. Amazing, awful, or just so-so: we want to hear what you have to say!

To receive your **FREE *PCCN Essential Test Tips* Video**, please email us at 5star@triviumtestprep.com. Include "Free 5 Star" in the subject line and the following information in your email:

1. The title of the product you purchased.
2. Your rating from 1 – 5 (with 5 being the best).
3. Your feedback about the product, including how our materials helped you meet your goals and ways in which we can improve our products.
4. Your full name and shipping address so we can send your FREE *PCCN Essential Test Tips* Video.

If you have any questions or concerns please feel free to contact us directly at 5star@triviumtestprep.com.

Thank you!

Table of Contents

Introduction

The PCCN certification is a designation provided by the AACN, granted to those who have demonstrated a thorough knowledge in progressive care nursing for acutely ill patients.

Who Should Take PCCN Exam?

The eligibility requirements for sitting in the PCCN exam include:

- Holding current licensure as an APRN or RN in the United States
- Meeting one of the following requirements regarding clinical practice:
  - Having practiced as an APRN or RN for 1,750 hours in direct bedside care of acutely ill adult patients during the previous two years. 875 of those hours must be completed in the year preceding applying for the exam.
  - Having practiced as an APRN or RN for a minimum of 5 years and of 2,000 hours care of acutely ill adult patients. 144 of those hours in direct bedside care must be in the year preceding applying for the exam.
- These credentials and hours may be subject to verification so that the AACN can verify clinical practice.

What is on the PCCN exam?

The PCCN exam lasts for 2 hours 30 minutes and has 125 items. However only 100 of them are scored. The other 25 questions are used for gathering information to improve future exams if needed. Approximately 80% of the exam will focus on "Clinical Judgment" and the other 20% will cover "Professional Caring and Ethical Practice". A majority of the exam focuses on age-specific patient groups, but some of it may also span across the entire average lifespan.

How to Apply

To apply for the PCCN, first ensure that you meet the requirements listed above, and then visit www.aacn.org to find more information and create and application. There is an exam fee of $175 if you are an AACN member, or $275 if you are not.

Chapter 1: Cardiovascular Disorders

ACUTE CORONARY SYNDROME: MYOCARDIAL INFARCTION

Any condition that is brought on by the sudden reduction of blood flow to the heart is referred to as an acute coronary syndrome, which is a life-threatening emergency. Myocardial infarctions occur when the coronary artery is suddenly occluded with a blood clot.

Myocardial infarctions are divided into two different types: ST segment elevation myocardial infarction (STEMI) and non-ST-segment elevation myocardial infarction (NSTEMI).

- Non-ST segment elevation myocardial infarctions (NSTEMI) are less severe than ST-segment elevation myocardial infarctions. This myocardial infarction occurs when a blood clot only partly occludes the artery. This partial occlusion results in partial heart muscle, rather than complete heart muscle, damage.

- ST segment elevation myocardial infarction (STEMI) occurs when the coronary artery becomes completely blocked. This results in the deterioration and death of almost all the heart muscles that are being supplied by the occluded artery.

Signs and Symptoms

The symptoms of acute coronary syndrome mimic those of a heart attack, and if not treated quickly, a heart attack will occur. The signs and symptoms are:

- Diaphoresis
- Dyspnea
- Nausea and vomiting
- Angina
- Referred pain

Prevention

Acute coronary syndrome can be prevented by maintaining heart health with a healthful diet, regularly exercising , abstaining from smoking, and having regular check-ups with a physician to check blood pressure and cholesterol levels.

Treatment

Depending on the symptoms and how severe the blockage is, a patient may be treated with the following medications:

- Aspirin
- Thrombolytics
- Nitroglycerin
- Angiotensin-converting enzymes
- Cholesterol-lowering drugs
- Calcium channel blockers
- Beta-blockers
- Angiotensin receptor blockers (ARBs)
- (Ace) inhibitors

In some cases, the medications are not enough to restore healthy blood flow through the heart. In these instances, surgery or other procedures such as angioplasty, stenting, or coronary bypass surgery may be necessary.

ACUTE INFLAMMATORY CARDIAC DISEASE

A bacterial or fungal infection of the endocardium can cause an acute inflammatory disease called endocarditis. This disorder can affect people of any age, but it is more prevalent in males than females. Additionally, those at greatest risk for endocarditis include patients who are immunocompromised and those who use illicit intravenous drugs.

The different classifications of infective endocarditis are:

- Acute bacterial endocarditis (ABE)
- Sub-acute bacterial endocarditis (SBE)
- Prosthetic valvular endocarditis (PVE)

Symptoms and Signs

The symptoms and signs of infective endocarditis depend on the classification of the endocarditis and its severity. Some of the signs and symptoms of sub-acute bacterial endocarditis are:

- Low-grade fever
- Night sweats
- Fatigue
- Malaise
- Weight loss
- Chills and arthralgias
- Tachycardia
- Pallor

The signs and symptoms of acute bacterial endocarditis and prosthetic valvular endocarditis include the same signs and symptoms listed above, but they tend to occur rapidly. Fever, heart murmurs, and septic shock may develop without warning. In very rare cases, purulent meningitis can occur.

Right-sided endocarditis can lead to septic pulmonary emboli, which is characterized by a cough, hemoptysis, tricuspid regurgitation murmur, and chest pain that is pleuritic in nature.

Treatment

The treatment for this disorder includes intravenous antibiotics and in some cases, valve debridement, repair, or replacement.

AORTIC ABDOMINAL ANEURYSM

An abdominal, or aortic, aneurysm occurs when the aorta's arterial wall is weakened and becomes abnormally dilated.

Signs and Symptoms

For the most part, aortic aneurysms do not present with any symptoms. However, as it worsens, the patient may experience pain and tenderness, or it may spontaneously rupture without any symptoms or warning.

Ruptured aneurysms usually present with back and abdominal pain, hypotension, and tachycardia.

Treatment

Treatment for aortic aneurysms depends on the size of an aneurysm. Small ones that do not enlarge over time may not require any treatment. Some aortic aneurysms enlarge, and others remain unchanged over time.

If an aneurysm ruptures, it is necessary for the patient to be treated immediately by surgery or endovascular stent grafting. Without immediate treatment, the mortality rate is 100%.

CARDIAC SURGERY

If all other treatments fail to work, cardiac surgery may be necessary. Coronary artery bypass grafting (CABG) is the most common type of cardiac surgery performed on adults. When coronary cardiac bypass grafting is performed, the surgeon takes a healthy artery or vein from the body and connects or grafts it to a blocked coronary artery.

Other cardiac surgeries are done to:

- Treat heart failure and coronary heart disease
- Control cardiac dysrhythmias
- Surgically replace the heart
- Repair damaged and abnormal structures of the heart
- Repair or replace a heart valve
- Implant a medical device, such as a pacemaker

Cardiac surgery usually has excellent results, but there are risks involved. Some of the risks are an infection, bleeding, irregular heartbeats, and stroke. Risks are greater in elderly women and among those with other diseases, such as peripheral arterial disease, lung disease, kidney disease, and diabetes.

CARDIAC TAMPONADE

Cardiac tamponade occurs when the pericardial sac rapidly collects fluid. The collection interferes with ventricular filling and contractions. This then causes a compression of the heart. Cardiac tamponade is a life-threatening medical emergency that requires immediate and rapid medical attention.

Risk Factors

The most common reasons for cardiac tamponade are:

- Breast, lung, or other cancers invading the pericardial sac
- The chest undergoing high levels of radiation
- A traumatic accident, such as an automobile accident, that causes a blunt force trauma to the chest
- Stab and gunshot wounds
- Hypothyroidism
- Pericarditis
- A ruptured aortic aneurysm
- An accidental puncture while placing a central line
- An accidental perforation during an angiography, pacemaker insertion, or cardiac catheterization
- Clogged chest drainage tubes

Symptoms and Signs

The symptoms and signs of cardiac tamponade include:

- Low urinary output
- Tachycardia
- Cool and mottled skin

- Paradoxical pulse
- Hypotension, narrowed pulse pressure, and weak peripheral pulses
- Distant and muffled heart sounds
- Decreased level of consciousness
- Jugular vein distention
- High central venous pressure

Treatment

This medical emergency requires hospitalization. Initially, the focus is on stabilizing the patient by relieving the pressure on the heart. The fluid in the pericardial sac needs to be drained, and this is usually done through a pericardiocentesis.

If a penetrating wound is present, the blood is drained, and clots are removed with a thoracotomy. There are occasions in which a portion of the pericardial sac is removed in order to relieve pressure on the patient's heart.

To return the patient's blood pressure to normal, oxygen, fluids, and medications may be necessary. Once the patient is stabilized, and the tamponade is under control, the treatment of any underlying conditions begins.

CARDIOGENIC SHOCK

Cardiogenic shock occurs when the patient's heart suddenly is not able to pump the amount of blood necessary to meet the needs of the body. The most common cause is a severe heart attack.

Cardiogenic shock is a rare condition, and if not treated immediately, can result in death. About 50% of those who develop cardiogenic shock can survive if treatment is administered immediately.

Signs and Symptoms

The signs and symptoms associated with cardiogenic shock include:

- Decreased urination
- Cold extremities
- Pale skin
- Sweating
- Weak pulse
- Fainting and loss of consciousness
- Confusion
- Tachycardia
- Severe shortness of breath
- Tachypnea

Prevention

Preventing heart attack is the best way to prevent cardiogenic shock, which includes:

- Controlling hypertension
- Quitting smoking
- Maintaining a healthful weight
- Lowering cholesterol and intake of saturated fats
- Exercising regularly

Complications

The complications of cardiogenic shock include organ damage, which can be permanent depending on how long the cardiogenic shock lasts, and death.

Treatment

Treating cardiogenic shock involves focusing repair on the damage to the heart muscles and other organs in the body that was caused by the lack of oxygen.

There are medications, medical procedures, and surgery that are available in the treatment of cardiogenic shock. Emergency life support, which may include mechanical ventilation, is often necessary.

The medications used to treat cardiogenic shock focus on improving the flow of blood to the heart and increasing the patient's heart pumping ability. Examples of these medications include:

- Aspirin
- Thrombolytics
- Superaspirins
- Heparin
- Inotropic agents

Procedures that can be used to treat cardiogenic shock by increasing blood flow through the heart are:

- Angioplasty and stenting
- Balloon pump

Surgery may be necessary to treat cardiogenic shock if other treatments are unsuccessful. Possible surgical interventions include:

- Heart transplantation
- Heart pumps

- Surgery to repair injury to the heart
- Coronary artery bypass surgery

CARDIOMYOPATHIES

Cardiomyopathies are primary disorders of the heart muscle that are divided into three types:

- Dilated cardiomyopathy:
  This type is a myocardial dysfunction that causes heart failure in which ventricular dilation and systolic dysfunction predominate.

  The symptoms associated with dilated cardiomyopathy include dyspnea, fatigue, and peripheral edema.

  Treatment focuses on correcting the cause of the dysfunction. If heart failure is severe and progresses, one of the following treatments may be necessary:

  - Heart transplant
  - Repair of moderate to severe valvular regurgitation
  - Implantable cardioverter-defibrillator
  - Cardiac resynchronization therapy

- Hypertrophic cardiomyopathy:
  This type can be congenital or an acquired disorder. It is characterized by marked ventricular hypertrophy including diastolic dysfunction, but it does not include increase afterload.

  This disorder can present with symptoms such as dyspnea, chest pain, syncope, and sudden death.

  Treatments include:

  - Beta-blockers
  - Verapamil
  - Disopyramide
  - Chemical or surgical reduction of outflow tract obstruction

- Restrictive cardiomyopathy:
  This type results from noncompliant ventricular walls that restrict the heart's diastolic filling. One or both sides of the heart can be affected, but the left side is the most commonly affected.

  The symptoms include fatigue and exertional dyspnea. Treatment can sometimes include surgery, but in most cases, it is unsuccessful.

CARDIAC DYSRHYTHMIAS

Sinus Bradycardia and Sinus Tachycardia

The normal heart rate is 60-100 beats per minute. Bradycardia is a slower than average heart rate (fewer than 60 beats per minute).

Sinus bradycardia occurs when the SA node takes longer than normal to depolarize as the result of some parasympathetic stimulation. The duration of diastole increases while the cardiac output decreases. This arrhythmia is often found among patients affected with coronary artery disease, during a myocardial infarction, secondary to increased intracranial pressure, and resulting from some medications such as digitalis and beta-blockers.

Some of the general signs and symptoms of bradycardia are:

- Fainting
- Weakness
- Dizziness
- Fatigue
- Shortness of breath
- Chest pain
- Confusion

The treatment depends on the cause, severity of the symptoms, and type of electrical conduction problem. Treatment choices include treatment of the underlying condition, a change in medication, and a pacemaker.

Tachycardia is a more rapid than normal heart rate (more than 100 beats per minute).

Sinus tachycardia occurs when the SA node depolarizes more quickly than normal. This dysrhythmia lowers coronary artery perfusion and cardiac output. The duration of diastole is shorter than that of a normal sinus rhythm.

Sinus tachycardia is associated with sympathetic nervous system stimulation such as occurs with strenuous exercise, stress, pain, hyperthyroidism, caffeine use, and cardiovascular response to hypovolemia and hypotension.

Some of the general signs and symptoms of tachycardia are:

- Palpitations
- Chest pressure or tightness
- Dizziness
- Lightheadedness

Like sinus bradycardia, the treatment of sinus tachycardia depends on the type of electrical conduction problem, the severity of symptoms, and the cause. Treatment choices include treatment of the underlying condition.

Sinus bradycardia and sinus tachycardia both have all the features of a normal sinus rhythm other than a standard rate of 60-100 beats per minute.

Atrial Flutter

Atrial flutter occurs when rapid atrial depolarization rates occur. The cardiac rate may be regular or irregular. The danger of thrombosis is present, but not to the extent that it can happen with atrial fibrillation.

Some of the causes of atrial flutter are heart failure, chronic pulmonary disease, and right-sided heart enlargement. When needed, this cardiac arrhythmia is treated with amiodarone, calcium channel blockers, beta-blockers, digitalis, and cardioversion.

Atrial Fibrillation

Atrial fibrillation is a relatively common arrhythmia among those affected by pulmonary embolus, hypoxia, a mitral valve disorder, and congestive heart disease, as well as among the elderly.

Cardiac output is decreased with this dysrhythmia. To prevent thromboembolism, emergency cardioversion may be indicated immediately after the administration of heparin or low molecular weight heparin.

Premature Atrial Contractions

Premature atrial contractions occur as the result of atrial cells taking over the role of the SA node. Normal QRS complexes occur, but the QRS is preceded by a premature P wave. This arrhythmia can result from a number of causes including nicotine, fatigue, alcohol, digitalis, electrolyte imbalances, ischemia, and hypoxia.

Paroxysmal Supraventricular Tachycardia

With this arrhythmia, the atria or the AV junction takes the pacemaker role from the body's natural pacemaker, which is the SA node. It usually appears and disappears in a rather rapid manner.

Some of the causes of paroxysmal supraventricular tachycardia are nicotine, caffeine, alcohol, stress, electrolyte imbalances, hypoxic episodes, and ischemia.

This cardiac arrhythmia is sometimes short-lived and self-limiting. Simple coughing or carotid massage may readily resolve it. Other treatment interventions include intravenous adenosine and cardioversion when the client is unstable as a result of this dysrhythmia.

First-Degree Atrioventricular Block

First-degree atrioventricular block occurs when the AV node impulse is delayed, thus leading to a prolonged PR interval. The P wave is present before each QRS complex.

It is very often asymptomatic, and treatment is typically not indicated unless the client is symptomatic. However, it should be noted that first-degree atrioventricular blocks can lead to more severe types of heart block.

Second-Degree Atrioventricular Block Type I

Second-degree atrioventricular (AV) block type I is also referred to as Wenckebach and Mobitz type I arrhythmias. This dysrhythmia is characterized by progressive delays of conduction through the AV node, which progressively lengthen the PR interval until it results in a missing QRS interval and a non-conducted P wave.

Again, treatment may not be necessary unless the client is symptomatic. Some cases may be caused by digoxin toxicity.

Second-Degree Atrioventricular Block Type II

Second-degree AV block type II, also referred to as Mobitz type II, occurs when the AV node impulses are intermittently blocked and do not reach the heart's ventricles. Second-degree AV block type II can lead to complete heart block. Treatment includes supplemental oxygen, intravenous atropine, and a temporary pacemaker.

Complete Heart Block (Third Degree Heart Block)

Third-degree heart block, or complete AV disassociation, occurs when no atrial impulses reach the ventricle, so a ventricular or junctional pacemaker takes over. This causes a lack of coordination between the ventricles and the atria and ventricles; the ventricular and atrial rates are different, and the QRS complex is wide.

Some of the risk factors associated with complete heart block are medications like beta-blockers and digoxin, a myocardial infarction, coronary heart disease, an atrial septal defect, and acute rheumatic fever.

The signs and symptoms include an altered level of consciousness, syncope, and chest pain.

Cardiac failure and cardiac arrest can occur as a result of this cardiac arrhythmia, so emergency treatment is necessary. Cardiac pacing should be started immediately, and preparation for basic and advanced life support should begin.

Premature Ventricular Contractions

Premature ventricular contractions are also referred to as extrasystole, premature ventricular complexes, and premature ventricular ectopic beats. It is a life-threatening emergency. Ventricular irritability causes abnormal impulses from an ectopic area in the ventricle. This life-threatening arrhythmia can be caused by electrolyte imbalances, acidosis, hypoxia, ischemia, and digitalis toxicity.

Premature ventricular contractions can occur in isolation (single focus) or clusters (multifocal). Multifocal patterns are called bigeminy and trigeminy, respectively. A couplet is two PVCs in succession, and a triplet is when three PVCs occur in succession.

Ventricular Tachycardia

NO cardiac impulses come from the atrium with life-threatening ventricular tachycardia. This arrhythmia often leads to ventricular fibrillation and asystole unless it is immediately treated.

The QRS complex is broadened, and the rate is dangerously fast and inefficient. Significant and life-threatening hemodynamic compromise occurs very rapidly.

Emergency interventions include cardioversion, intravenous lidocaine and magnesium sulfate, and antiarrhythmic medications such as amiodarone.

Ventricular Fibrillation

Ventricular fibrillation occurs when there are chaotic and rapid signals from ectopic ventricular sites. All of the ventricular contractions are ineffective; therefore, no cardiac output occurs. Death is very likely when this arrhythmia persists for more than six minutes.

The treatment involves immediate advanced life support including defibrillation, intravenous adrenaline, and 100% supplemental oxygen. A lack of treatment leads to asystole.

Asystole

Asystole, or a flat line, is the total and complete absence of any ventricular activity despite the fact that atrial impulses and P-waves may be present.

Immediate advanced life support is necessary. Intravenous adrenaline, sodium bicarbonate, and atropine, as well as 100% oxygen, are done in hopes of saving the person's life.

GENETIC CARDIAC DISEASE

Genetic heart disease, such as long QT and Brugada syndromes, are inherited, and as such, cannot be prevented. They often affect more than one family member.

Long QT Syndrome

Long QT syndrome affects the heart rhythm and can lead to tachycardia, fainting, and seizures. At times, it can result in sudden death.

Signs and Symptoms

Long QT syndrome can appear as early as one month of age or can be postponed until middle-age. Some people will not experience any symptoms, but possible symptoms include:

- Fainting
- Seizures
- Sudden death

Prevention

Inherited long QT syndrome symptoms and complications can be precipitated by certain medications such as decongestants, appetite suppressions, antibiotics (erythromycin), and illicit street drugs like amphetamines and cocaine.

All of these precipitating medications should be avoided.

Treatment

Treatment can include medications such as beta-blockers, mexiletine, fish oil, and potassium.

Other interventions can include a pacemaker, left cardiac sympathetic denervation surgery, and lifestyle changes like healthful nutrition and regular exercise.

Brugada

Brugada is a potentially life-threatening disorder that is commonly an inherited genetic disorder. It is a heart rhythm disorder, in which there are abnormal heartbeats called a Brugada sign.

Signs and Symptoms

In the majority of cases, Brugada presents with no symptoms, but with an ECG, the irregular pattern is seen. Some possible symptoms are syncope, irregular heartbeats, and palpitations. It can lead to sudden cardiac arrest.

Treatment

The most commonly used treatment is an implantable cardioverter defibrillator.

HEART FAILURE

Heart failure can be chronic or acute. The greatest risk factor for heart failure is age. The incidence and prevalence of heart failure increases with advanced age.

Simply stated, heart failure is the lack of the heart's ability to pump enough oxygenated blood to meet the demands and requirements of the body's tissues. Pathophysiologically, neural, renal, hemodynamic, and hormonal responses occur as the result of heart failure.

Some of the most common causes of heart failure include cardiomyopathy, hypertension, and ischemic heart disease. Left ventricular systolic compromise is the most common underlying cause of heart failure, but right-sided ventricular dysfunction, as well as biventricular failure, can also cause it.

Signs and Symptoms

This lack of oxygenation can lead to a number of signs and symptoms including fatigue, fluid retention (edema), dyspnea, tachycardia, pallor, lethargy, activity intolerance, weakness, and anxiety.

Other signs and symptoms of heart failure can include the following:

- Chest pain
- Difficulty concentrating
- Rapid or irregular heart rate
- Lack of appetite and nausea
- Ascites

Prevention

To prevent heart failure, it is necessary for the patient to change certain lifestyle choices. Prevention measures include smoking cessation, regular exercise, healthful diet, stress management, as well as controlling blood pressure, cholesterol, and diabetes.

Complications

Complications of heart failure depend on the cause, the severity, the patient's age, and the patient's overall health. Some complications include:

- Damage or failure of the kidneys
- Damage to the liver
- Stroke
- Heart valve problems

Heart failure can be life-threatening; however, with treatment, some people can improve. Therefore, emergency care is necessary for all patients.

Treatment

Depending on the symptoms and severity of the heart failure, there are several options for treatment. Medications such as ACE inhibitors, digoxin, beta-blockers, diuretics to reduce fluid overload, inotropes, aldosterone antagonists, and angiotensin II receptor antagonists are used. Other medications such as anticoagulants to prevent clotting, nitrates for chest pain, and other medications to treat the symptoms are sometimes necessary.

More invasive treatments include:

- Replacement or repair of a heart valve
- Coronary bypass surgery
- Heart pumps
- Heart transplantation
- Implanted cardioverter defibrillators (ICDs)

Finally, it is recommended that the patient have restricted fluid intake, a low-sodium diet, and a medically approved exercise routine.

HYPERTENSIVE CRISIS

A hypertensive crisis occurs when a patient has a dramatically high increase in blood pressure of 180 mm Hg over 120 mm Hg or higher. Hypertensive crisis is a life-threatening emergency.

Symptoms and Signs

The symptoms and signs of a hypertensive crisis include:

- Seizures
- Shortness of breath
- Severe anxiety

- Unresponsiveness
- Nausea and vomiting
- Severe chest pain
- Severe headache, which can be accompanied by blurred vision and confusion

Treatment

Treatment for hypertensive crisis includes hospitalization, oral or intravenous antihypertensive drugs, and other emergency procedures, as indicated.

Chapter 2: Pulmonary Disorders

ACUTE RESPIRATORY DISTRESS SYNDROME

Acute respiratory distress syndrome (ARDS) is the build-up of fluid in the alveoli in the lungs. The fluid in the lungs takes away from the space that can be filled with oxygen, therefore depriving the organs of the body of oxygen.

Acute respiratory distress syndrome is more prevalent among those who are critically ill or those who have been injured.

Symptoms and Signs

The symptoms and signs of acute respiratory distress syndrome include:

- Low blood pressure
- Breathing that is labored and rapid
- Confusion
- Lethargy
- Severe shortness of breath

Risk Factors

The majority of people who develop acute respiratory distress syndrome do so in the hospital because they are usually chronically ill people. Alcoholics are also at risk for developing this syndrome.

Complications

Acute respiratory distress syndrome is an extremely serious disorder with a high mortality rate. Some of the possible complications are the risk of infections, abnormal lung function, blood clots, pneumothorax, pulmonary fibrosis, and cognitive dysfunctions including memory loss and depression.

A severe type of acute respiratory distress syndrome, known as acute lung injury, has been used as an umbrella term for hypoxic respiratory failure, which is a serious condition that occurs when the cells in the body are unable to receive a sufficient amount of oxygen.

Acute lung injury is caused by any and all systematic inflammation, which includes sepsis. Other causes of acute lung injury include:

- Pneumonia
- Major trauma
- Radiation

- Poisoning
- Eclampsia
- Air embolism
- Amniotic fluid embolism
- Massive blood transfusion
- Fat embolism
- Inhalation of noxious fumes
- Burns
- Pulmonary aspiration and near drowning

Treatment

Immediate treatment includes the monitoring and support of the patient's ABCs. Supplemental oxygen and mechanical ventilation are often needed.

Medications are also used in the treatment of patients with acute respiratory distress syndrome. These drugs are used to minimize gastric reflux if present, prevent any possible clots from forming in the legs and lungs, prevent and treat infections, and help ease any pain.

EXACERBATION OF COPD

Chronic obstructive pulmonary disease (COPD) exacerbation means that there is a sudden worsening of the COPD symptoms. The symptoms most common with COPD, such as coughing, dyspnea, and sputum production, are worsened.

Symptoms and Signs

The symptoms and signs of an exacerbation of COPD include increased breathlessness and:

- Fever
- Wheezing
- Tightness in the chest
- Sputum color and thickness change
- Increased coughing and sputum production

Prevention

There are certain things that can be done in order to prevent an exacerbation of COPD including adhering to the medication regime; getting an annual flu and pneumonia vaccine, which can help to decrease severe illness and death for COPD patients by as much as 50%; good hygiene such as hand washing; maintaining a balanced diet; exercise; eight hours of uninterrupted sleep; avoiding air pollution/smoking and crowds of people, especially during the flu season.

The top two causes of COPD exacerbations are respiratory infections (bacterial and viral) and air pollution.

Treatment

Depending on the condition of the patient, possible treatments can include:

- Oxygen therapy
- Ventilation by either mask or intubation
- Respiratory stimulants
- Bronchodilators
- Antibiotics, if there is an underlying bacterial infection
- Glucocorticosteroids (oral, intravenous, or inhaled) to treat inflammation

OBSTRUCTIVE SLEEP APNEA

Obstructive sleep apnea is a disorder in which a patient, while asleep, stops and starts breathing repeatedly. This continues throughout all sleep sessions. The reason for this apnea is the relaxation of the oral and throat muscles, which blocks the patient's airway, therefore causing the cessation of breathing.

This is the most common type of sleep apnea. It can affect anyone, but in most instances, it affects middle-age and elderly people who are overweight. In studies, men with this disorder are at risk of heart failure, whereas women are not.

Signs and Symptoms

The most common symptom of obstructive sleep apnea is snoring, and in most cases, the snoring is quite loud. Other signs and symptoms include:

- Daytime lethargy and narcolepsy
- Intermittent apnea
- Abrupt awakening during sleep with shortness of breath or gasping
- A dry mouth, sore throat, headache, and chest pain upon awakening
- Hypertension
- Insomnia
- Irritability
- Depression
- Difficulty with concentration

Complications

Obstructive sleep apnea is a serious medical condition with a number of complications. Some of these complications threaten the patient's health, whereas other symptoms can be considered a mere annoyance to others, like snoring.

Some of the complications include:

- Cardiovascular problems: Hypertension, arrhythmias, hypoxia or hypoxemia, increased risk of heart failure, heart attack, coronary artery disease, heart disease, and stroke.

- Medication and surgical complications: Medications such as narcotic analgesics and sedatives can lead to increased apnea because they tend to relax the upper airway; surgical patients may experience respiratory problems during and after surgery.

- Excessive fatigue: This fatigue can lead to physical, psychological, and social impairments. Narcolepsy can be dangerous because the affected patient can fall asleep while driving an automobile, for example.

Treatment

Patients who experience more mild cases of apnea can benefit from lifestyle changes such as exercise, weight loss, smoking cessation, use of nasal decongestants, and not sleeping on their back.

Other options for obstructive sleep apnea include:

- Therapies such as CPAP for mild to moderate cases
- Medications to decrease daytime drowsiness
- Surgery or other procedures such as uvulopalatopharyngoplasty (UPPP), jaw surgery (maxillomandibular advancement), tracheostomy, implants known as the Pillar procedure, nasal surgery to remove polyps, and surgery to remove tonsils and/or adenoids

PULMONARY EMBOLISM

A pulmonary embolism is a sudden blockage in one or more of the lung arteries, caused by blood clots from somewhere else in the body. The blood clot, in most cases, is from the leg as the result of deep vein thrombosis. The clot breaks loose and travels through the bloodstream to the lungs. This is a serious life-threatening condition, which can cause permanent damage to the affected lungs and other organs in the body and death.

Risk factors associated with pulmonary embolism include:

- Increased coagulation factors such as II, VII, VIII, and X
- Increased production of fibrin
- Decreased fibrinolytic activity

- Increased resistance to protein C

- Decreased free protein S levels

The Signs and Symptoms

Shortness of breath coupled with tachycardia is very suggestive of a pulmonary embolus. Other signs and symptoms include:

- Chest pain
- Weak pulse
- Irregular heart beat
- Coughing
- Hemoptysis
- Tachypnea
- Hypotension
- Cyanosis
- Syncope
- Diaphoresis
- Skin pallor
- Wheezing

Diagnosis

A chest X-ray has limited usefulness in terms of diagnosis. It is, however, helpful for ruling out other causes of respiratory compromise particularly when done in conjunction with arterial blood gasses and an electrocardiogram. Doppler ultrasound of both lower limbs can detect deep vein thrombosis, and a definitive diagnosis requires the use of scanning using ionizing radiation or magnetic resonance imaging.

The Complications

This serious pulmonary disorder can lead to respiratory failure, pleural effusion, pulmonary infarction, hemorrhage, and death.

Prevention

Some prevention strategies can include:

- Pneumatic compression to promote venous return
- Compression stockings to promote venous return
- Anticoagulation therapy when indicated
- Physical activity and mobility
- Therapeutic and preventive exercises

The Treatment

Immediate emergency interventions include the provision of airway and oxygenation needs with supplemental oxygen to maintain an oxygen saturation of at least 95%.

Later treatment includes anticoagulation therapy to prevent reoccurrence and to limit the growth of existing clots. These medications do NOT dissolve existing clots. Intravenous heparin and low molecular weight heparin are used. In an emergency, protamine sulfate reverses the effects of the heparin. Warfarin is given concurrently with, and after, heparin therapy to prevent pulmonary emboli. A vena cava filter may also be inserted when indicated.

PULMONARY HYPERTENSION

Pulmonary hypertension is a dangerous type of blood pressure illness. It affects the lungs and the right side of the heart. This illness, if not treated appropriately and effectively, can be life-threatening.

Symptoms and Signs

The symptoms and signs of pulmonary hypertension, in its early stages, can be unnoticeable and asymptomatic for months or even years. Once the disease progresses and becomes more serious, however, the symptoms can become noticeable and severe.

Some symptoms that the patient may experience include:

- Syncope
- Dyspnea
- Fatigue
- Edema in the ankles and legs, which can eventually result in ascites
- Heart palpitations
- Tachycardia
- Cyanosis
- Pain or pressure in the chest

Complications

Some of the complications include:

- Cor pulmonale
- Blood clots, which are most common in the small arteries in the lungs
- Arrhythmias, some of which can be life-threatening
- Bleeding into the lungs, causing coughing up blood and life-threatening hemorrhage and respiratory compromise

Treatment

The treatment of pulmonary hypertension is quite extensive. In addition to supplemental oxygen and respiratory support, some of the medications used include:

- Vasodilators
- Anticoagulants
- High-dose calcium channel blockers
- Sildenafil and tadalafil
- Diuretics

Surgical interventions can include heart or lung transplant and open heart atrial septectomy.

RESPIRATORY FAILURE

Respiratory failure is a condition that occurs when there is not enough oxygen passing from the lungs into the blood or when the lungs are unable to remove enough carbon dioxide from the blood. High levels of carbon dioxide and low levels of oxygen occur simultaneously.

Respiratory failure can be acute, which develops quickly and is an emergency medical condition, or chronic, which develops slowly and lasts for a longer period.

Signs and Symptoms

Respiratory symptoms and signs can vary depending on the underlying cause, whether it is acute or chronic, and the levels of carbon dioxide and oxygen in the blood.

When there is a low oxygen level in the blood, the patient can experience shortness of breath and a feeling of being unable to get enough air, no matter how he/she breathes. When oxygen levels are severely low, the patient will have a bluish, cyanotic coloring of the skin, fingernails, and lips. If the carbon dioxide level in the blood is high, the patient may be confused and may hyperventilate.

Other symptoms can include sleepiness, loss of consciousness, and cardiac arrhythmias.

Complications

Some of the complications associated with respiratory failure include hypoxia, which, if severe, can lead to anoxia. If anoxia is left untreated, it can result in tissue loss, multisystem failure, and death.

These patients, who most often require mechanical ventilation when respiratory functioning is significantly compromised, are also at risk for ventilator-related complications such as:

- Nosocomial infections

- Deep vein thrombosis
- Pressure ulcers
- Gastritis and ulcers
- Pulmonary embolism
- Hypotension
- Acute respiratory alkalosis
- Pneumonia

Treatment

The primary goal is to oxygenate adequately the patient.

The specific treatments used are:

- Oxygen therapy
- Ventilator support
- Tracheostomy
- Fluids
- Medications
- Treatment of underlying cause

RESPIRATORY INFECTIONS

A respiratory infection can be chronic or acute, and it can be an upper respiratory infection or a lower respiratory infection.

Upper respiratory infections, more frequent than lower respiratory ones, affect the nose, sinuses, pharynx, or larynx. Examples of upper infections are tonsillitis, sinusitis, otitis media, the common cold, etc. Lower respiratory infections affect the lower respiratory tract, which includes the trachea, airways, and lungs. Some examples are bronchitis, croup, and pneumonia.

Signs and Symptoms

Upper respiratory infections include these symptoms:

- Sore throat
- Headache
- Sneezing
- Stuffy or runny nose
- Muscle aches
- Pressure in the face
- Nasal congestion
- Coughing up blood

Signs and symptoms of lower respiratory infections can include:

- Fatigue
- Headache
- Wheezing
- Sore throat
- Stuffy nose
- High fever
- Body aches
- Chest tightness
- Sinusitis
- Loss of breath

PNEUMONIA

Pneumonia, which is a common type of respiratory infection, is a lung infection caused by bacteria or viruses. The risk of pneumonia increases with immune system compromise, as can occur when the patient has a cold or flu and/or chronic disorder like asthma, heart disease, chronic obstructive pulmonary disease, or diabetes.

Signs and Symptoms

Signs and symptoms can include:

- Fever
- Cough
- Tachycardia
- Chest pain
- Diarrhea
- Nausea and vomiting
- Lethargy
- Chills accompanied by shaking

Prevention

For people over 65 years of age, people who smoke, and people who have a heart or lung disorder, it is strongly recommended that they get a pneumococcal vaccine. The vaccine does not always prevent pneumonia, but it does prevent it from being as severe a case if it is contracted.

Other helpful tips are to keep good hygiene, which includes washing hands often, because it helps avoid the spread of viruses and bacteria and to avoid people who have the flu, measles, chicken pox, or even the common cold.

Treatment

Antibiotics will be used if the cause is bacterial. If a virus causes the pneumonia, antibiotics are usually not given, but they can be used to treat some bacterial complications that may arise.

Rest, taking care of the symptoms (such as taking cough medicine for a cough), not smoking, and drinking plenty of liquids is the usual course of treatment. More complicated and severe cases need supportive treatment with fluid monitoring and replacement and respiratory monitoring and support.

Tuberculosis (TB)

Tuberculosis is transmitted by the airborne inhalation of the tubercle bacilli. The inflammatory process and cellular reaction creates a small, firm, white nodule called a primary tubercle, the center of which contains the bacilli. Cells gather around this center, and the outer portion becomes fibrosed.

This infectious disease often lays dormant for years with no ill effects or symptoms. However, with some physical or emotional stress, the bacilli start to multiply, causing destruction of lung tissue and possible mortality. Most healthy people who are exposed to TB do not develop active disease, but X-ray evidence does show a calcified nodule called a Ghon tubercle.

Signs and Symptoms

The clinical manifestations of TB include:

- Low-grade fever
- Pallor
- Chills
- Night sweats
- Fatigability
- Anorexia
- Weight loss
- Productive cough
- Purulent, blood-stained sputum
- Dyspnea late in the disease process
- Localized chest pain

TB is diagnosed with the tuberculin PPD skin test (Mantoux), sputum smears, cultures, and a chest x-ray examination. A positive skin test reaction does not confirm the active disease, but just that the patient has developed antibodies to the infectious agent.

The most threatening complication of TB is the development of an untreatable drug-resistant strain of TB; patients with TB must consistently continue their medication regimen to prevent drug resistance. Compliance poses many challenges, particularly when poverty and homelessness are present.

The pharmacological treatment of tuberculosis is based on individual needs and the results of susceptibility testing. Some of the medications used to treat TB include INH, rifabutin, rifapentine, pyrazinamide, rifampin, ethambutol, streptomycin, capreomycin, aminosalicylate sodium, cycloserine, and ethionamide.

Combination therapy, rather than a single medication, is the most effective form of treatment.

Mononucleosis

Infectious mononucleosis is an acute disease caused by the Epstein-Barr virus. The highest incidence is among young adults between 15 and 30 years of age. Mononucleosis is self-limiting with recovery after 2-3 weeks.

It presents with flu-like symptoms of malaise, headache, general aches, fever, fatigue, sore throat, pains, spleen enlargement, and lymphadenopathy. Rare and severe clinical manifestations include rupture of the spleen and encephalitis.

The blood count will show increased mononuclear leukocytes and a total white cell count of 10,000-20,000/mm^3.

Treatment

The patient recovers in 2-3 weeks with rest and acetaminophen. Resuming full or strenuous activities should not be attempted for 4-6 weeks, however.

Rubeola (Measles)

The rubeola virus is transmitted by contact and airborne droplets of infectious material from respiratory tract secretions, blood, or urine of an infected person. The incubation period is 8-20 days, and it is communicable during the prodromal (catarrhal) stage from 4-5 days before the appearance of the rash.

Symptoms and Signs

The symptoms and signs include fever, malaise, coryza, cough, conjunctivitis, Koplik spots, and a erythematous maculopapular rash that starts on the face and spreads to the body followed by desquamation.

Complications

Some of the complications include pneumonia, otitis media, bronchiolitis, obstructive laryngitis, and encephalitis.

Treatment

The treatment is supportive with rest, isolation until after the fifth day of the rash, fluids, fever management, cool mist for cough and coryza, and a darkened room for photophobia.

Rubella (German Measles)

The rubella virus is transmitted by airborne droplets, direct contact with infectious droplets, and indirect contact with nasopharyngeal secretions, fecal, and urine.

The incubation period ranges from 14-21 days, and it is communicable from 5-7 days before the rash appears.

Symptoms and Signs

The symptoms and signs include headache, malaise, lymphadenopathy, fever, sore throat, cough, coryza, and a rash that begins on the face and spreads in a downward manner to the neck, shoulders, trunk, and legs. With resolution, the rash regresses in an upward manner.

Complications

The complications of rubella include rare arthritis, encephalitis, and purpura. The greatest danger associated with rubella is its teratogenic effects on a developing fetus.

Treatment

The treatment is primarily supportive, comfort, and isolation from pregnant women.

Varicella

Varicella, also known as Chickenpox, is caused by the herpes varicella-zoster virus. The incubation period ranges from 14-21 days, and it is communicable from 1 day before the appearance of the rash and up to 6 days after the vesicles have crusted.

Transmission occurs by direct contact, droplets, and contaminated objects (fomites).

Symptoms and Signs

The symptoms and signs of varicella include malaise, anorexia, low-grade fever, an extremely pruritic rash on the trunk and scalp, and lesions on the mucous membranes of the perineal area and oral cavity.

Treatment

Strict isolation precautions must be followed to prevent both airborne and contact transmission. Other interventions include supportive care, skin care (topical calamine lotion), keeping fingernails short or mittened if the child is scratching, teaching the child to put pressure on itchy areas rather than scratching, and avoiding aspirin.

Respiratory Syncytial Virus (RSV)

RSV is a highly communicable upper respiratory infection that commonly causes bronchiolitis accompanied with the production of thick mucus, which can occlude the bronchioles.

Symptoms and Signs

The symptoms and signs include the production of thick mucus, cough, ear infection, pharyngitis, tachypnea, cyanosis, fever, respiratory stridor, wheezing, listlessness, hypercapnia, and periods of apnea in severe cases. Respiratory failure is a serious complication associated with RSV.

Treatment

The treatment of RSV includes supportive care, antibiotics if a bacterial infection is suspected, symptom management (humidity, rest, and fluids), intravenous fluid replacement, O_2, and other respiratory treatments. Aspirin is not used because of the risk of Reye's syndrome.

Influenza

Influenza is a viral infection that disrupts the respiratory system. Influenza can cause a mild to severe illness depending on who it affects. More serious complications can affect vulnerable populations such as young children, pregnant women, older adults, those with weakened immune systems, and those with chronic illnesses.

Signs and Symptoms

The signs and symptoms can range from mild to severe including a painful, productive cough; malaise; hoarseness; photophobia fever; and myalgia. Symptoms usually persist for 4-5 days although some patients can remain symptomatic for a week or more.
Complications

The most severe and serious complications associated with this infection include encephalitis; acute viral hemorrhagic pneumonia; and secondary bacterial infections such as pneumonia, bronchitis, otitis media, and sinusitis.

Although healthy people should experience no complications or less severe complications such as bronchitis a, they will feel horrible for a brief period.

Signs and Symptoms

Influenza can cause cold-like symptoms, but unlike a cold, influenza comes on strong and suddenly.

Common signs include:

- Headache
- Fever over 100° F
- Chills and sweats
- Aching muscles
- Nasal congestion
- Fatigue and weakness
- Dry cough

Prevention

The Centers for Disease Control and Prevention recommends that everyone in the United States over six months of age receive an annual flu vaccination. The vaccine each year is made to protect from the three most common types of flu viruses for that year. It can be given by injection or nasal spray.

Other tips for preventing this virus are to keep good hygiene, which includes washing hands frequently and covering coughs and sneezes and to avoid large crowds, particularly during the influenza season.

Treatment

In most cases, bed rest and plenty of fluids are the only treatment necessary. Antiviral medications such as Tamiflu or Relenza may be given to help prevent serious complications from occurring; they also can help shorten the duration of the virus by a day or two. Care and treatment are generally supportive and includes fever management, fluids, rest, and symptomatic relief. Aspirin should NOT be given because of the risk of Reye's syndrome.

Meningitis

Meningitis is an inflammation of the meninges' pia layers and the cerebrospinal fluid. The causative pathogens can be a virus, bacteria, or fungi including streptococcus pneumoniae, group B streptococcus, haemophilus influenzae, neisseria meningitis, staphylococci and gram-negative organisms like escherichia coli, serratia, and enterobacter. Meningitis is often a life-threatening, medical emergency.

Symptoms and Signs

The symptoms and signs of meningitis include fever, headache, nuchal rigidity, altered mental status (particularly among the elderly), petechial or puerperal rash, and arching of the back and neck. Children and infants may refuse feeding and have a blank stare, seizures, photophobia, and positive Brudzinski's and Kernig's signs. Infants may have bulging fontanels.

Encephalitis

Encephalitis is the inflammation of the cerebral tissue, and viral infection is most often its cause. Acute viral encephalitis is caused by herpes simplex among children, and adults may experience postischemic inflammatory encephalitis as a complication of a cerebrovascular accident. The West Nile virus, cytomegalovirus, and toxoplasma can also cause encephalitis.

Symptoms and Signs

Some of the symptoms and signs include fever, disorientation, motor weakness, seizures, headache, altered neurological functioning, nausea, vomiting, and bizarre behavior.

Treatment of Meningitis and Encephalitis

Meningitis and encephalitis are treated with seizure precautions, maintaining a quiet environment, medications, assessing and monitoring vital signs and neurological status frequently, reorienting the person, administering antipyretics as needed, monitoring fluids, and measuring intake and output.

SEVERE ASTHMA

Severe asthma can be a life-threatening condition.

Signs and Symptoms

The symptoms of a severe asthma attack are similar to those of respiratory system failure. These symptoms are:

- Constant shortness of breath
- Breathlessness that is not relieved by lying down
- A need to stand up to breathe more easily

- A feeling of the chest being closed
- Unable to speak full sentences
- Lips appearing bluish in color
- Hunched shoulders
- Strained abdominal and neck muscles
- Agitation, confusion, and inability to concentrate

Treatment

Severe asthma attacks are treated with respiratory therapies such as a nebulizer and medications such as epinephrine, corticosteroids, magnesium sulfate, leukotriene, and injections of terbutaline. These drugs aim to reduce inflammation.

If the severe asthma attack does not respond to any of those treatments, it may be necessary to use a mechanical ventilator to ensure adequate oxygenation.

THORACIC SURGERY

Thoracic surgery is chest surgery that is performed to treat disorders of the chest or lungs such as lung cancer, emphysema, gastroentroesophageal reflux, mesothelioma, pleural diseases, and many others.

A lobectomy is the removal of a lobe of the lung. A lobectomy is commonly used to treat lung cancer. The entire lobe of the lung is removed to excise the tumor, in addition to the surrounding tissue, when the tumor is relatively small.

After the surgery, the patient usually requires a chest tube to drain fluids; mechanical ventilation and oxygen may also be required.

A pneumonectomy is a surgical procedure that removes the entire lung. It is the surgery of choice when other options for treating lung cancer are not working. It is also the operation of choice when a patient has had a traumatic chest injury in which there has been severe damage to the bronchus and/or major blood vessels in the lung that cannot be repaired and when a tumor is located near the center of the lung. Lung cancer patients, as well as COPD patients, are usually the most common pneumonectomy patients.

Chapter 3: Endocrine, Hematological, Gastrointestinal, and Renal Disorders

ENDOCRINE SYSTEM DISORDERS

DIABETES MELLITUS

Diabetes mellitus is the most common disease of the endocrine system. It is a chronic systematic disease that alters the protein, carbohydrate, and fat metabolism.

TYPE I DIABETES MELLITUS

Type 1 diabetes mellitus, also called insulin-dependent diabetes, is a chronic condition that results when the pancreas does not produce insulin, or it provides an insufficient amount.

Genetics and exposures to certain viruses, among other factors, can contribute to type 1 diabetes.

Symptoms and Signs

Some of the symptoms and signs include blurry vision, frequent urination, excessive hunger and thirst, lethargy, and weight loss.

Complications

Type I diabetes can damage the body's major organs like the heart, kidneys, eyes, blood vessels, and nerves, particularly when blood glucose is not controlled. Some of the most severe complications include renal damage; neuropathy; gastroparesis; heart disease; stroke risk; vascular damage; diabetic retinopathy; blindness; cataracts; glaucoma; poor peripheral microcirculation, which can lead to limb loss; infection; diabetic coma; and death.

Treatment

The ultimate goal of treatment is the control of blood glucose levels. This control is achieved with insulin, diet, and exercise.

TYPE 2 DIABETES MELLITUS

Type 2 diabetes, also called adult-onset diabetes, is a chronic condition that can occur from insulin resistance or the lack of adequate insulin production. Currently, the U.S. is seeing many children developing type 2 diabetes despite the fact that it is referred to as adult onset diabetes.

Signs and Symptoms

Many people live with this type of diabetes for years without knowing they are affected by it. The signs and symptoms are identical to those described above for type 1 diabetes. The etiology and pathophysiology of these symptoms are described below:

- Excessive thirst and frequent urination: Results from excessive sugar in the bloodstream, which causes fluid to be pulled from the tissues.

- Hunger: This occurs when the amount of insulin cannot move glucose into the cells for energy. Energy depletion leads to hunger.

- Weight loss: This occurs because the body cannot metabolize glucose.

- Fatigue: Energy is depleted when glucose metabolism is disrupted.

- Impaired healing: Diabetes affects the body's ability to heal and resist infections.

- Blurry vision: High glucose levels pull fluid from the eyes' lenses.

Prevention

Type 2 diabetes can be prevented with healthful lifestyle choices like a healthy diet, weight management, and daily exercise. People with prediabetes can help ward off the development of diabetes by changing their diet and exercise; those who already have been diagnosed with diabetes can prevent serious complications from occurring by following the same healthful choices.

Some preventive strategies include reducing weight if indicated; eating healthy foods such as low calorie and low fat foods; incorporating fruits, whole grains, and vegetables into the diet; and exercising daily for half an hour, which can consist of walking, swimming, biking, etc.

Complications

The complications of diabetes can affect virtually all bodily organs and functions and can be life-threatening. Some of these complications are heart and blood vessel disease, neuropathy, nephropathy, diabetic retinopathy, osteoporosis, and recurring infections.

Treatment

Type 2 diabetes is treated with a combination of weight management, diet, exercise, oral hypoglycemic medications, and insulin, when necessary.

GESTATIONAL DIABETES

Gestational diabetes is a type of diabetes that can be developed during pregnancy, and like other forms of diabetes, it affects how the cells in the body use glucose. This kind of diabetes is a danger to both the mother and the child. Gestational diabetes usually resolves after the birth of the baby; however, type 2 diabetes continues to be a risk for women with a history of gestational diabetes throughout their lives.

Signs and Symptoms

There may be no noticeable signs or symptoms of gestational diabetes, but occasionally, the pregnant woman may experience excessive thirst and/or increased frequency and amount of urination.

Prevention

Some healthful choices for women planning on getting pregnant or those who are already pregnant are eating nutritious foods such as high-fiber and low-fat/calorie foods like fruits, vegetables, and whole grains; consistently exercising on a daily basis; and losing excess weight before pregnancy.

Complications

The majority of women with gestational diabetes give birth to healthy babies, but if the diabetes is not carefully watched and the blood sugar levels are not controlled, there can be complications to both the child and the mother, the most common of which is an emergency C-section.

Some examples of complications that can affect the baby are excessive birth weight, pre-term birth, respiratory distress syndrome, jaundice, future type 2 diabetes and obesity, and death.

Some examples of complications that can affect the pregnant woman are the development of type 2 diabetes, hypertension, preeclampsia, and eclampsia, some of which can be life-threatening.

Treatment

Treatment includes regular blood sugar monitoring; a healthful diet; medications like insulin or an oral hypoglycemic agent such as glyburide, when indicated; and regular exercise. Exercise is helpful for managing weight and increasing the sensitivity of the cells to insulin; it also relieves pregnancy-related muscle cramps, back pain, swelling, constipation, and sleeping problems.

DIABETIC KETOACIDOSIS

Diabetic ketoacidosis is one of the serious complications that can occur from diabetes. This disorder leads to the buildup of ketones, a toxic acid, in the bloodstream. It is a life-threatening emergency.

Symptoms and Signs

The symptoms and signs of diabetic ketoacidosis can present very quickly and without warning. Some of the initial signs and symptoms are a fruity breath odor, fatigue, weakness, nausea, vomiting, shortness of breath, abdominal pain, and confusion.

Hyperglycemia and high ketone levels in one's urine are more specific signs, and they can be easily detected through an at-home blood and urine test. Untreated diabetic ketoacidosis can be fatal, so it is pertinent to seek emergency care immediately if one experiences multiple symptoms, if ketones are present in the urine, and/or if the blood glucose level is higher than 300 mg/dL.

Prevention

To prevent diabetic ketoacidosis, there are a number of things that should be done. These include managing the diabetes, which entails maintaining a healthful diet, regular exercise, and keeping up with doctor visits; monitoring blood glucose levels; adjusting insulin as needed; and checking ketone levels regularly.

If diabetic ketoacidosis is suspected, emergency care should be sought right away.

Complications

The possible complications of diabetic ketoacidosis are hypoglycemia, hypokalemia, and cerebral edema. This is a dangerous disorder; if left untreated, it can lead to coma and even death.

Treatment

Treatment of diabetic ketoacidosis typically takes place in the hospital and includes:

- Fluid replacement, which can be either oral or intravenous, to help rehydrate and flush excessive glucose out of the blood.

- Electrolyte replacement, which is given intravenously, because the absence of insulin can lower many of the body's electrolytes.

- Insulin therapy, which reverses the hyperglycemic processes that caused diabetic ketoacidosis.

DIABETIC HYPERGLYCEMIC HYPEROSMOLAR SYNDROME (HHS)

Diabetic hyperglycemic hyperosmolar syndrome (HHS) is a disorder in which a patient's blood glucose levels is very high without the presence of ketones. This is a complication of type 2 diabetes.

Signs and Symptoms

Among the signs and symptoms are less major ones like weight loss, weakness, nausea, lethargy, increased thirst, increased urination, fever, and confusion. Some of the more life-threatening and severe signs and symptoms are convulsions, coma, and speech impairments.

Prevention

Preventing this life-threatening endocrine disorder involves the control of type 2 diabetes and recognition of the early signs of both dehydration and infection.

Complications

Some of the possible complications associated with this disorder are acute circulatory collapse, the formation of blood clots, cerebral edema, and lactic acidosis.

Treatment

Treatment's ultimate goal is to correct the patient's dehydration. Intravenous fluids and potassium are necessary, and intravenous insulin will help treat the high glucose levels in the blood.

HYPOGLYCEMIA

Hypoglycemia is a severe, life-threatening disorder that affects many diabetic clients taking insulin or oral diabetes hypoglycemic agents.

Symptoms and Signs

The symptoms and signs of hypoglycemia include:

- Excessive hunger
- Diaphoresis
- Anxiety
- Shakiness
- Heart palpitations
- Double or blurry vision
- Confusion
- Seizures
- Loss of consciousness

Prevention

Hypoglycemia can be prevented with the correct balance of diet, exercise, and medication. For example, hypoglycemia can occur as the result of too much strenuous exercise, too little to eat, and too much insulin or oral hypoglycemic agent.

It can be prevented by eating small amounts of food throughout the day rather than three large meals to maintain steady blood glucose levels, by decreasing the medication dosage when strenuous exercise is anticipated, and by carefully monitoring blood glucose levels.

Complications

If the signs and symptoms of hypoglycemia are not treated for a period, the person can lose consciousness, experience seizures, and lapse into a coma because of the lack of glucose, which is needed to allow the brain to function properly, among other things.

Treatment

The treatment of hypoglycemia begins with the rapid raising of the blood glucose level. Conscious patients can ingest candy, fruit juice, or glucose tablets. Most diabetics are encouraged to carry glucose tablets with them in case of such a situation, especially early on in the disease since the precise balance of insulin, diet, and exercise is not yet established. Unconscious clients cannot take anything by mouth; therefore, glucagon must be administered parenterally.

METABOLIC SYNDROME

Metabolic syndrome is a group of conditions that occur together. This group of conditions includes high blood glucose level, high blood pressure, abnormal cholesterol levels, and an excess of body fat around the waist. Metabolic syndrome increases the risk of diabetes, stroke, and heart disease.

Symptoms and signs

Three or more of the following symptoms can be indicative of metabolic syndrome:

- High cholesterol: Triglycerides of 150 mg/dL or more and the high-density lipoprotein cholesterol of less than 40mg/dL for men and less than 50 mg/dL for women
- High blood glucose levels: A fasting blood glucose level of 100 mg/dL or more
- High blood pressure: A diastolic blood pressure of 85 mm Hg or higher or a systolic blood pressure of 130 mm Hg or higher
- Obesity around the waist: A waist circumference of 35 inches or more for women and 40 inches or more for men

Prevention

Preventing metabolic syndrome involves preventing one or more of the conditions that make up this syndrome. In order to do so, it is important to maintain a healthful diet, which should include eating fruits, vegetables, and lean meat such as chicken and should avoid fried foods and excessive amounts of red meat and salt. Regular exercise, regular check-ups, and an optimal blood glucose level are also preventive measures about which the patient should know.

Complications

The complications of metabolic syndrome include the risk of diabetes, cardiovascular disease such as a heart attack, and cerebrovascular accident, or stroke.

Treatment

The treatment of metabolic syndrome consists of treating all of the conditions that make up this disorder. It takes an aggressive change in the patient's lifestyle to treat this syndrome. In some cases, medications are used to treat one or more of the underlying conditions. A reduction in weight, blood pressure, cholesterol, and blood glucose levels are all necessary in the treatment of metabolic syndrome. To achieve these, a daily exercise routine, weight loss program, change in diet, and smoking cessation are necessary.

HEMATOLOGICAL SYSTEM DISORDERS

Anemias

Anemia is a condition in which there are not enough healthy red blood cells in the body to carry sufficient oxygen to the tissues in the body. There are various forms of anemia, of which the loss of blood is the most common. Anemia can range from mild to severe, and it can also be temporary or permanent.

Signs and Symptoms

The various forms of anemia have several signs and symptoms associated with them. At first, the signs may be slight, but as the anemia gets worse, the symptoms will progress as well. The symptoms do vary based on the cause, but some of the signs and symptoms include a headache, cool or cold extremities, alterations of cognitive functioning, dizziness, fatigue, shortness of breath, chest pain, tachycardia, irregular heartbeat, and pale skin.

Prevention
Types of Anemia and Treatments Available

TYPE OF ANEMIA	TREATMENT OPTIONS
Iron Deficiency Anemia	Dietary changes Iron supplements Stopping any bleeding Possible surgery
Vitamin Deficiency Anemia	Dietary supplements Increased dietary nutrients Vitamin B-12 injections
Chronic Disease Anemia	No treatment for anemia Treatment of underlying disease Blood transfusion or injections of erythropoietin
Aplastic Anemia	Blood transfusions Bone marrow transplantation
Anemias Associated with Bone Marrow Disease	Medication Chemotherapy Bone marrow transplantation
Hemolytic Anemia	Treatment depends on the type and cause • Blood transfusion • Plasmapheresis • Drugs to suppress the immune system may be used when an overactive immune system causes the hemolytic anemia • Supplemental folic acid and iron are used to replace losses when the

	blood cells are being destroyed at a faster rate than production • Splenectomy
Sickle-Cell Anemia	Oxygen Pain relief drugs Blood transfusions Folic acid supplements Antibiotics Bone marrow transplantation Hydroxyurea, which is a cancer drug Oral and IV fluids for pain and prevention of complications
Thalassemia	Blood transfusions Folic acid supplements Bone marrow transplantation Splenectomy

CANCER

Chemicals, radiation, and viruses are external risk factors related to cancer; internal or intrinsic risk factors include hormones, chemotherapy drugs, genetics, and immune system alterations. The following list includes the most common risk factors for cancer:

- Age:
  Most cancers occur in people who are over the age of 65. Nonetheless, persons of all ages, including young children and young adults, can also be impacted by cancer, but the older age group is most prone.

- Tobacco Use:
  Tobacco use is the most preventable of all cancer risk factors and cancer deaths. Regular use of tobacco products dramatically increases the risk of getting cancer.

  Smokers are more likely than non-smokers to develop cancer in the larynx, mouth, bladder, lungs, esophagus, kidney, pancreas, cervix, and throat. They are also more likely to develop acute myeloid leukemia.

- Sunlight:

Sunlight is another avoidable risk factor. The sun's ultraviolet (UV) radiation causes aging of the skin and skin damage that may lead to skin cancer. Medical professionals recommend that people of all ages limit their time in the sun, use sunscreen, and avoid other sources of UV radiation such as sunlamps and tanning booths.

- Ionizing Radiation:
  Ionizing radiation is considered an environmental risk factor associated with cancer. Ionizing radiation comes from rays that enter the earth's atmosphere from outer space, radioactive fallout, radon gas, x-rays, therapeutic radiation for cancer, and other sources. Ionizing radiation can cause cell damage, which leads to cancer.

- Chemicals and Other Substances:
  Many studies have shown that exposure to asbestos, benzene, benzidine, cadmium, nickel, and vinyl chloride may cause cancer. Asbestos exposure is a well-established risk factor for malignant mesothelioma.

- Pathogens Including Viruses and Bacteria:
  Between 1985 and 2005, scientists found that evidence could demonstrate approximately 15% of the world's cancer deaths can be traced to parasites, bacteria, or viruses. Some of these bacteria and viruses include human papillomavirus (HPV), which is associated with cancer of the cervix, vagina, penis, anus, and mouth and hepatitis B and C, which are associated with liver cancer. The Helicobacter pylori places one at risk for cancer of the stomach, and the Epstein-Barr virus is associated with Burkitt's lymphoma.

- Hormones:
  Hormone therapy has been, in the past, an ongoing standard of treatment for menopausal women. Currently, hormone replacement therapy has much more limited use in terms of the duration and frequency of treatment than it did in the past. Hormones are also used for the treatment of some cancers, like cancer of the prostate and breast. This hormonal treatment of cancer can lead to other cancers. The types of cancer that are most commonly associated with this include prostate, breast, and uterine cancer.

- Family History: Genetics and Familial Tendency:
  Certain types of cancers such as uterine, ovarian, and breast cancer reoccur throughout generations of family members. A few types of cancers (colon and early-onset breast cancer) have been linked to tracked, familial genes. Therefore, inheriting certain genes may increase a person's susceptibility to particular cancers.

- Occupational and Avocational Risks:
  Some occupations and hobbies can place people at risk for many illnesses and disorders including cancer. For example, construction and demolition workers may be exposed to asbestos, and some hobbies like chemistry may pose a risk in terms of chemical exposure.

- Alcohol:
  The excessive consumption of alcohol has been linked to certain types of cancer (liver). When alcohol consumption and tobacco use are combined, the chances of developing the disease significantly increase.

- Being Overweight, Lack of Physical Activity, Poor Diet:
  It is estimated that about 35% of all cancers are related to dietary causes. Excessive eating and the lack of regular physical activity and exercise leads to obesity, which is associated with cancers of the uterus, ovary, gall bladder, prostate, pancreas, rectum, colon, and breast. Being inactive and overweight are also risk factors for cancers of the uterus, kidney, esophagus, colon, and breast.

The Signs and Symptoms

The signs and symptoms, as well as the diagnosis, of cancer, depend on the type of cancer and the site of cancer. Some diagnostic procedures include laboratory testing including testing for tumor markers, biopsies, and diagnostic imaging like x-rays; computerized tomography (CT) scans; ultrasonography; magnetic resonance imaging (MRI) and nuclear medicine imaging (a two-dimensional image, or 2D scintigraphy); and a three-dimensional image, or 3D scintigraphy.

The Treatment of Cancer

The four major categories of cancer treatment are surgery, chemotherapy, radiotherapy, and biotherapy. Surgical intervention is the oldest and the most common treatment for cancer.

In the past, surgery was the only option for treatment of cancer, but now, surgery as the primary treatment occurs in only about 60% of oncology cases. Surgery, however, is also used for a number of other reasons, in addition to cure. It is used to diagnose cancer (biopsy) among most clients, to stage cancer, for prophylaxis, to palliate symptoms, to reconstruct bodily parts, and to prevent and control some oncological emergencies.

Radiation can be used to destroy the tumor, ensure that surrounding tissue and lymph nodes are free of cancer, reduce pain, shrink the tumor, and relieve an obstruction. Radiation kills cells, especially those in faster-growing tumors and tissues. Radiation can kill the quickly multiplying cancer cells, but over time, radiation can also kill the healthy cells. Ideal radiation therapy reduces or eliminates cancer without any damage to the normal surrounding tissue.

Radiation therapy can be broadly categorized as external or internal. External radiation is applied to the body with a linear accelerator that delivers electron and gamma ionizing radiation for a minute or so, as based on the prescribed dosage, depth of the tumor, and type of radiation beam being used. External radiation is also referred to as teletherapy.

Internal radiation, or brachytherapy, which is also referred to as internal, interstitial, or intracavity radiation, delivers the radiation in high doses into the tumor by temporarily placing the radioactive material directly into or next to the tumor. It can be sealed with a seed, wire, or needle, and it can also be unsealed in the form of an oral or systemic preparation.

Brachytherapy is used for cancers like those affecting the cervix, endometrium, rectum, breast, prostate, lungs, esophagus, head, and neck. Special radiation precautions are initiated with brachytherapy to protect visitors and healthcare providers from the harmful effects of the radiation.

Chemotherapy drugs include:

- Alkylating drugs
- Antimetabolites
- Antitumor antibiotics
- Mitotic inhibitors
- Hormones
- Biotherapy also referred to as immunotherapy or biological response modifier therapy

HEMOSTASIS DISORDERS

Disseminated Intravascular Coagulation (DIC)

This disorder occurs as a result of several underlying conditions and diseases. It does not occur as a primary condition; it is always secondary to some other condition or illness. This disorder is unique and somewhat paradoxical. It affects thrombosis, or clotting, as well as bleeding. There is a lack of balance between anticoagulation and coagulation.

Risk Factors

Some of the risk factors associated with DIC, in addition to cancer, are:
- Hepatic disease
- Hypoxia
- Infections, especially gram-negative sepsis
- Hypersensitivity reactions
- Vascular disorders
- Pregnancy

Neoplastic acute leukemia, pheochromocytoma, and adenocarcinoma are most often associated with disseminated intravascular coagulation.

Signs and Symptoms

The chronic form of disseminated intravascular coagulation has a slow onset over weeks or months, and it leads to excessive clotting without bleeding. Acute DIC occurs rapidly, and it is marked with excessive clotting and then severe bleeding.

Other signs and symptoms can include a headache; tachycardia; hypotension; changes in mood, behavior, and level of consciousness; and peripheral cyanosis secondary to microvascular thrombosis.

Interventions

The nonpharmacological and pharmacological interventions aim to prevent life-threatening complications, such as impaired perfusion and death, to maintain tissue and organ perfusion and to eliminate the cause, if possible.

Specific interventions include the administration of blood products like fresh frozen plasma and packed red cells to replace clotting factors and fluids. Hypoxia, acidosis, and hypotension are corrected, and recombinant human activated protein C may be administered.

Nursing Implications

Nurses must closely assess for bleeding, fluid overload as the result of fluid/blood replacements, and urinary and renal compromise. Hourly urines are collected to evaluate cardiac and renal perfusion and functioning.

Drug-Induced Thrombocytopenia: Heparin and Other Drugs

Platelet destruction can develop as the result of immunological and nonimmunological causes. For example, viral infection, drugs, blood transfusions, and connective tissue or lymphoproliferative disorders are examples of immunologic causes. Sepsis and acute respiratory distress syndrome are examples of nonimmunological causes of thrombocytopenia.

The Symptoms and Signs

Some of the symptoms and signs include mucosal bleeding, purpura, and petechiae. Laboratory findings depend on the cause.

Some drugs that are commonly used can occasionally induce thrombocytopenia. They include heparin, quinine, trimethoprim/sulfamethoxazole, glycoprotein IIb/IIIa inhibitors, hydrochlorothiazide, carbamazepine, acetaminophen, vancomycin, chlorpropamide, ranitidine, and rifampin. Heparin-induced thrombocytopenia (HIT) can result from even a very low dose of heparin.

Immunosuppressive Disorders Associated With Thrombocytopenia

- HIV infection may cause immunologic thrombocytopenia
- Hepatitis C
- Systemic viral infections like Epstein-Barr virus and cytomegalovirus, rickettsial infections such as bacterial sepsis and Rocky Mountain spotted fever

Sepsis often causes nonimmunologic thrombocytopenia such as that which occurs with disseminated intravascular coagulation, the formation of immune complexes that can associate with platelets, platelet deposits on damaged endothelial surfaces, and platelet apoptosis.

GASTROINTESTINAL DISORDERS

Some functional gastrointestinal disorders include obstructions, ileus, diabetic gastroparesis, gastroesophageal reflux, and irritable bowel syndrome.

Obstruction

An obstruction of the intestinal region is a blockage that keeps food or liquid from passing through the small or large intestine. Obstructions can be caused by adhesions formed after surgery, diverticulitis, hernias, and tumors.

Treatment for obstructions does depend on the cause of the blockage, but in most cases, it requires hospitalization.

Paralytic Ileus

Paralytic ileus is defined as hypomotility of the gastrointestinal tract in the absence of any mechanical bowel obstruction. Patients usually experience mild pain in the abdominal region and also some bloating. In some cases, they can also experience vomiting, nausea, and loss of appetite.

Most cases occur as the result of intra-abdominal surgery and anesthesia. Once the treatment of the underlying disease is addressed, the paralytic ileus will diminish.

Diabetic Gastroparesis

Diabetic gastroparesis is a condition in which the stomach of the patient is unable to function normally; the patient is not able to empty the stomach properly. It interferes with the patient's digestive system and can cause nausea and vomiting as well as problems with blood sugar.

The cause of diabetic gastroparesis is unknown; it is thought to be caused by some type of nerve damage. Although there is no cure for diabetic gastroparesis, it is important to control the patient's blood glucose level.

Gastroesophageal Reflux

Gastroesophageal reflux, commonly referred to as GERD, is a chronic digestive disease. GERD occurs when a patient experiences reflux, which is the occasional flow of bile and digestive acids into the esophagus that irritates the lining of the esophagus.

The signs and symptoms are heartburn and acid reflux. If the patient experiences these symptoms more than two or three times a week, it is GERD. GERD is usually easy to treat with over-the-counter medication, but some may need prescription-strength medications or, in more severe cases, surgery.

Irritable Bowel Syndrome

Irritable bowel syndrome is an extremely uncomfortable and embarrassing disorder for many people. The patient may experience chronic abdominal pain, bouts of uncontrollable diarrhea, and constipation.

There are both prescription and over-the-counter medications that can be used to treat the symptoms of this syndrome and make the patient more comfortable. Psychotherapy and stress management therapy are also alternative treatment methods for irritable bowel syndrome. The good news is that this condition does not and will not lead to any further complications.

Ischemic Colitis

Ischemic colitis is a disease that occurs when there is a decrease in blood flow to the colon due to narrowed or blocked arteries. The reduced blood flow deprives the digestive system of sufficient oxygen. This disorder can cause pain and can also damage the patient's colon. It can affect any part of the colon, but in most cases, the pain is reported on the left side of the abdomen.

This disease is most commonly seen in persons 60 years of age or older. Often, this is misdiagnosed because it presents very similar to other digestive conditions.

Signs and Symptoms

There is a variety of signs and symptoms that patients with ischemic colitis can experience. Possible symptoms include:

- Pain, which can be located in any part of the abdomen and can come on suddenly or gradually
- Bowel urgency
- Discolored stool, which can be bright red in color or more dull-like
- Passage of blood, which can occur instead of a bowel movement
- Diarrhea

If the pain is on the right side of the abdomen, it may be a sign of a more severe problem like a blockage of the small intestine since the arteries that feed the right side of the colon also supply part of the small intestine. It can lead to the life-threatening condition of necrosis, which is a loss of the intestinal tissue. Surgery is often necessary to clear the blockage and to remove the part of the intestine that has been damaged.

Prevention

Preventive measures for a person at risk for ischemic colitis include:

- Treatment of the underlying condition, which can be diabetes, heart disease, or high blood pressure
- Medication to lower cholesterol
- A daily exercise program
- Avoidance of medications that reduce blood flow

Complications

Most cases of ischemic colitis resolve on their own within a few days, but there are more severe cases, which can have the following complications:

- Ischemic stricture, which is a bowel obstruction
- Segmented ulcerating colitis, which is bowel inflammation
- Perforation of the intestine
- Persistent bleeding
- Gangrene due to the decreased blood flow and ischemia

Treatment

Depending on the severity of the condition, the treating physician may recommend antibiotics, which will prevent any infections from occurring; intravenous fluids if the patient is dehydrated; treatment for any underlying conditions such as congestive heart failure or a cardiac arrhythmia; or not taking medications that could possibly constrict the blood vessels such as migraine drugs, hormone medications, and some drugs that are prescribed for the heart.

In severe cases, when there is damage to the colon, surgery may be necessary. The operation can include removing ischemic tissue, repairing any perforation of the colon, bypassing the intestinal artery, and removing part of the colon. Surgery is more likely for those who have an underlying condition such as heart disease or low blood pressure.

Gastrointestinal (GI) Bleeding

Gastrointestinal (GI) bleeding is a definitive sign that there is a problem in the digestive tract. GI bleeding can occur in any of the gastrointestinal organs including the stomach, esophagus, colon or large intestine, small intestine, rectum, and the anus.

Upper GI bleeding is bleeding in the esophagus, stomach, or small intestine, whereas lower GI bleeding is bleeding in the large intestine, rectum, or anus.

Symptoms and Signs

Although the symptoms and signs of GI bleeding can vary, they usually include:

- Dark black, tar-like stool, which indicates an upper GI tract bleed
- Bright red stool, which can indicate a lower GI bleed
- Vomiting blood
- Ground coffee-like vomit
- Paleness
- Weakness
- Shortness of breath

Causes

In the upper GI tract, a common cause of bleeding is peptic ulcers, which are sometimes caused by a bacterial infection. Other conditions that can lead to upper GI bleeding include esophageal varices and Mallory-Weiss tears, which are tears in the walls of the esophagus. The most common cause of lower gastrointestinal bleeding is colitis. Other causes are Chron's disease, parasites, food poisoning, infections, and hemorrhoids.

Treatment

Treatment for gastrointestinal bleeds includes:

- Gastric lavage and suctioning
- Blood transfusions
- IV fluids and medications

Gastrointestinal Infections

Gastrointestinal (GI) infections occur when a virus, bacteria, or parasite infects a part of the GI tract. These types of infections are most common in the intestines and are the most common cause of GI food poisoning.

Bacterial infections include salmonella, shigella, and E-coli. Some infections caused by parasites are giardia and cryptosporidium. Viral GI infections, which are also referred to as gastroenteritis and the stomach flu, are most commonly caused by the rotavirus and noroviruses. These viral infections are highly contagious.

Symptoms and Signs

Some of the common symptoms and signs of GI infections are:

- Stomach cramps
- Nausea
- Fever
- Loss of appetite
- Bloody stool
- Dehydration

The duration of a GI infection depends on some factors such as the type of infection, the overall health of the person affected, etc. Viral and bacterial infections usually last between two and ten days.

Treatment

The majority of viral and bacterial infections do not require any treatment, but parasite infections may need to be treated with anti-parasitic medication.

HEPATIC FAILURE

Hepatic failure, also known as liver failure, occurs when large parts of the liver become damaged beyond repair, which renders the liver unable to function. This is a life-threatening emergency that can happen quickly, as is the case with acute liver failure; more commonly, however, it occurs gradually over several years, as is the case with chronic hepatic failure.

Signs and Symptoms

Often, liver failure is hard to diagnose because the early symptoms are similar to those of other conditions. Early symptoms include:
- Lethargy
- Nausea

- Diarrhea
- Loss of appetite

As liver failure progresses, the signs and symptoms become more severe, and they require immediate emergency care. The more severe symptoms include:

- Hepatic encephalopathy (confusion and disorientation)
- Easy bleeding and bruising
- Jaundice
- Swollen abdomen
- Drowsiness
- Coma

Prevention

Preventive measures of cirrhosis and hepatitis, as shown below, can prevent hepatic failure:

- Hepatitis vaccine or immunoglobulin shot to prevent hepatitis A and B

- Protective sexual activities, which means using condoms for all sexual activity including oral, anal, and vaginal

- Hand washing, which is essential to prevent the spread of germs

- Healthful diet, which includes eating plenty of fruits and vegetables, as well as other food groups

- Alcohol in moderation

- Avoiding acetaminophen (Tylenol)

- Not handling blood or other bodily fluids without using protective gloves

- Not sharing personal hygiene items such as razors or toothbrushes

Treatment

If liver failure is the result of a virus, the patient can be given supportive care to treat the symptoms, in the hospital, to allow the virus to run its course. In cases like this, the liver usually recovers on its own.

In severe cases, where there has been long-term deterioration, initially, the goal is to try to save whatever part of the liver is still functioning, but if this is not possible, a liver transplant is necessary. Liver transplants are relatively common and have an excellent rate of success.

PANCREATITIS

Pancreatitis is an inflammation of the pancreas. There are both acute and chronic forms of this disorder. Some cases can be mild and cured with lifestyle changes; in other cases, pancreatitis can be a serious condition with possible life-threatening complications.

Symptoms and Signs

The symptoms and signs of pancreatitis vary considerably. Acute pancreatitis is marked with:
- Nausea
- Vomiting
- Abdominal pain (upper abdomen), which increases after ingesting food
- Abdominal tenderness
- Pain that radiates from the abdomen to the back

Chronic pancreatitis can present with these symptoms:

- Steatorrhea
- Weight loss (without trying)
- Upper abdominal pain
- Indigestion

Complications

The complications associated with pancreatitis are quite serious:

- Pancreatic cancer
- Kidney failure
- Pseudocyst
- Malnutrition
- Infection
- Diabetes
- Breathing problems

Treatment

The initial treatment of pancreatitis is focused on reducing the inflammation of the pancreas. Treatment includes pain medication because of the severe pain caused by this disorder, abstaining from eating so that the pancreas has an opportunity to recover, and intravenous fluids to keep the body hydrated.

The treatment varies depending on the underlying cause:

- Cholecystectomy if the cause of the pancreatitis is gallstones
- Pancreatic surgery either to drain the fluid from the pancreas or to remove any diseased tissue that may be present
- Alcohol dependence treatment, when indicated, when excessive drinking is the causative factor
- Removal of any bile duct obstruction

Other treatments include pain management and oral pancreatic enzyme supplementation.

MALNUTRITION

Malnutrition can occur if one does not get enough nutrients—protein, carbohydrates, fats, vitamins, and minerals. Malnutrition compromises and jeopardizes physical and mental health. In severe cases, death can occur.

There are two types of malnutrition: a failure to thrive and malabsorption disorders.

Failure to Thrive

Failure to thrive describes children who do not receive or are unable to utilize, retain, or take in the calories required for them to gain the weight they need to grow as expected. Crucial periods of mental and physical development occur within the first few years of life, and it is during this period where most of the diagnoses of failure to thrive are made.

Permanent mental development can occur in a child who is not given the necessary nutrients he/she needs in the first year of life because this period is when the brain grows and develops the most. During the first year of life, the brain grows as much as it will during the rest of the person's life.

Physical development is also affected when proper nutrients are not received. Kids with failure to thrive are usually unable to meet physical milestones, whereas children without it can. For example, most babies will double their birth weight within the first four months of their life and triple that weight by the time they are one-year-old.

Signs and Symptoms

Some symptoms of failure to thrive include avoiding eye contact; irritability; loss of interest in their surroundings; and not reaching developmental milestones such as sitting up, crawling, walking, talking, etc.

There are many reasons why one may suffer from failure to thrive, and they include:

- Social factors, which include not feeding a child enough due to poverty, not wanting the child to get fat, neglect, distractions, or forgetting to feed the child

- Gastrointestinal problems, which include celiac disease, chronic liver disease, cystic fibrosis, chronic diarrhea, and gastroesophageal reflux disease (GERD)

- Chronic illness or medical disorder, which can include different types of cancers or other serious diseases, cleft lip or palate, or a premature baby

- Infections, which include parasites, urinary tract infections, and tuberculosis; they can force the body to expend excessive amounts of energy and also can cause a loss of appetite

- Metabolic disorders, which can limit the ability of the body to make use of all of the calories it ingests because of an inability to break down foods into energy

Treatment

The treatment for the failure to thrive depends on the underlying cause of this disorder. For example, for a child who is experiencing difficulties feeding, such as problems with breastfeeding latching, a nursing coach can be helpful, as can an occupational and speech therapist can use his/her expertise in the muscular control that is necessary for eating, and can help the mother and child with sucking and/or swallowing problems. If the failure to thrive is due to a disease or disorder, it may be necessary to consult with a specialist such as a cardiologist, neurologist, gastroenterologist, etc.

When the failure to thrive is related to a caregiver's neglect or similar issue, a social worker and, in some cases, another mental health professional like a psychologist can be involved in order to address the situation and ensure the child is given the proper nutrients he/she needs in order to live a healthy life. High caloric foods or formulas are often recommended.

More severe cases may require a feeding tube that can provide the child with a steady amount of nutrition. In extreme cases, a child may need to be hospitalized for feeding and close monitoring.

Malabsorption Disorders

Malabsorption occurs when disorders disorder interfere with food digestion or directly with nutrition absorption, malabsorption occurs. Disorders that involve the prevention of adequate food mixing of stomach acid and digestive enzymes adversely affect digestion, as is the case when the patient has had a partial or complete gastrectomy.

Other causes include a lactase deficiency; decreased digestive enzyme production; decreased bile; increased digestive acid production; and other insults to the gastrointestinal system including infections, drugs (such as cholestyramine, tetracycline, colchicine, and alcohol), and disorders (such as celiac disease, Chron's disease, intestinal wall lymphoma, and an inadequate supply of blood to the small intestine).

Symptoms

The most common symptom is chronic diarrhea. Steatorrhea results from inadequate fat absorption in the digestive tract. Flatulence, abdominal bloating, and explosive diarrhea can all result from inadequate absorption of sugars.

Deficiences of all nutrients or selective dificiences of sugars, proteins, fats, and minterals can be the result of malabsorption.

Weight loss, edema, dry skin, hair loss, anemia, fatigue, and weakness can occur.

RENAL DISORDERS

ACUTE RENAL FAILURE

When the kidneys are suddenly unable to filter waste products from the blood, this is called acute renal failure, more commonly referred to as acute kidney failure. This condition develops quickly, and when the kidneys lose their ability to filter, a dangerous level of waste accumulates in the body.

This condition normally affects those who are critically ill, and it can be life-threatening. If it occurs in a healthy person, it can be reversed, and normal kidney function can be restored.

Signs and Symptoms

There are several signs and symptoms that are associated with acute renal failure, but in some cases, the symptoms are not noticed until laboratory blood tests are processed. Some of the signs and symptoms are:

- Fatigue
- Drowsiness
- Shortness of breath
- Nausea
- Chest pain and pressure
- Confusion
- Decreased urine output
- Fluid retention; particularly dependent edema

Prevention

There is no exact way to prevent kidney failure, but taking good care of the kidneys can always help reduce the risk. Maintaining a healthful lifestyle and drinking alcohol only in moderation are helpful. When using over-the-counter medications, it is important to follow the instructions and not take too high of a dose because they can adversely affect the kidneys. It is also important for people with diabetes and high blood pressure to control and manage these chronic disorders.

Complications

Some potential complications include:

- Muscle weakness related to fluid and electrolyte imbalances
- Chest pain when the pericardial area is affected
- Fluid buildup, which can lead to shortness of breath and other respiratory complications
- Permanent kidney damage and loss of function in end-stage renal disease
- Death

Treatment

The treatment of acute kidney failure depends on the cause. The treatment involves the identification of and treatment for the underlying illness or injury that damaged the kidneys.

CHRONIC KIDNEY FAILURE

Chronic kidney failure is the gradual loss of function of the kidneys that can lead to dangerous alterations of bodily fluids, electrolytes, and waste buildup in the body.

Symptoms and Signs

The symptoms and signs of chronic kidney failure include:

- Decreased cognitive functioning
- Muscular twitching and cramps
- Hypertension that is sometimes difficult to control
- Chest pain
- Shortness of breath
- Decreased urinary output
- Fatigue and weakness
- Sleeping problems
- Hiccups
- Nausea

- Vomiting
- Anorexia
- Edema
- Persistent itching

Prevention

Some ways to help reduce the risk of chronic kidney failure are to:

- Reduce alcohol intake
- Maintain a healthful weight
- Maintain a healthy lifestyle
- Cease smoking
- Avoid the use of acetaminophen and other nephrotoxic medications
- Visit the doctor regularly

Complications

Survival of irreversible renal damage (end-stage kidney disease) requires either a kidney transplant or dialysis. Other complications include:

- Cardiovascular disease
- Decreased immune response
- Infection
- Pericarditis
- Hyperkalemia, which can be life-threatening
- Central nervous system alterations including poor concentration, confusion, personality changes, and seizures
- Impotence and decreased sexual drive
- Anemia
- An increased risk of bone fractures and weakened bones
- Pregnancy complications that potentially harm the developing fetus and mother
- Fluid retention, which can lead to edema, hypertension, and pulmonary edema

Treatment

The ultimate goal of chronic kidney failure treatment is to slow the progression of the kidney damage. This can be achieved by controlling the underlying cause. Often dialysis and transplantation are the only treatments for chronic kidney failure, but depending on its underlying cause, some types of chronic kidney failure can be treated.

Treatment of chronic kidney failure focuses on treating the signs and symptoms to slow the disease's progression and reduce complications. If the kidneys become severely damaged, it may be necessary for the patient to receive end-stage treatments for the kidney disease. Chronic kidney disease can progress to end-stage kidney disease, a fatal diagnosis in the absence of a kidney transpant or dialysis.

CONTRAST-INDUCED NEPHROPATHY

Radiopaque contrast agents are often used in radiography and fluoroscopy studies. These contrast agents are iodine-based. Many have severe adverse effects including allergic reactions and contrast nephropathy, which can lead to renal damage.

In some patients, intravascular injection of an iodinated contrast agent causes serum creatinine to increase transiently. Most of these patients have no symptoms and recover all normal renal functioning in less than one week. However, some develop chronic kidney disease.

Some of the risk factors associated with contrast-induced nephropathy include:

- Elevated creatinine, which indicates renal impairment
- Hypertension
- Heart failure
- Diabetes mellitus
- Multiple myeloma
- 70 years of age and older
- Use of nephrotoxic drugs

Prevention

Some cases can be prevented with the use of a reduced dosage of the contrast, the use of iso-osmolality agents, and hydration with the intravascular administration of 0.9% normal saline at 1 mL/kg for 24 hours beginning a couple of hours prior to the use of the contrast material.

END-STAGE RENAL DISEASE

End-stage renal disease (ESRD), commonly referred to as end-stage kidney disease, is the complete, or just about complete, shutdown and failure of the kidneys.
Signs and Symptoms

There are various signs and symptoms of end-stage renal disease. Some of the signs and symptoms, in addition to the ones described above for chronic renal disease, include:
- Abnormally dark or light skin
- Nail changes
- Bone pain
- Numbness in the extremities
- Breath odor
- Easy bruising

- Nosebleeds
- Bloody stool
- Excessive thirst
- Frequent hiccups
- Edema
- Vomiting, especially in the morning

Prevention

To prevent end-stage renal disease, the treatment of chronic kidney disease must be completed successfully. In some cases, this treatment is not effective, and death is imminent.

Complications

There are many complications associated with the end-stage renal disease. These include:

- Coronary artery disease
- Skin dryness and itching/scratching, which can lead to infection
- Seizures
- Hepatic failure
- Hyperkalemia
- Anemia
- Gastrointestinal bleeding
- Stroke
- Pericarditis
- Malnutrition
- Changes in blood glucose
- High levels of phosphorus
- Bone, joint, and muscular changes

Treatment

In addition to symptom relief, the only treatments for this disorder are dialysis and a kidney transplant.

ELECTROLYTE IMBALANCES

Electrolyte imbalances include potassium, calcium, magnesium, and sodium imbalances in the bloodstream.

Signs and Symptoms

The signs and symptoms for each electrolyte in excess and in deficit are distinctly different from imbalances of other electrolytes. Nonetheless, the general symptoms that may occur with an electrolyte imbalance include:

- Fatigue
- Nausea without vomiting
- Dizziness
- Trembling
- Constipation
- Dark urine
- Decreased urine output
- Muscle weakness
- Stiff or aching joints
- Dry skin
- Dry mouth
- Bad breath
- Poor elasticity of the skin
- Sunken eyes

Serious symptoms include tachycardia and changes in mental status.

Prevention

Aside from immediate treatment for the imbalance, it is vital that the cause of the imbalance be determined and treated. Possible causes include kidney disease, hormone/endocrine problems, stomach disorders, improper diet, loss of bodily fluids due to illness, and side effects of chemotherapy or medications. For example, some of the drugs that can lead to electrolyte imbalances are steroids, tricyclic antidepressants, birth control pills, diuretics, cough medicines, laxatives, steroids, and excessive amounts of antacids.

Complications

Some potential complications include:

- Shock
- Hyperthermia
- Cerebral edema
- Seizures or convulsions
- Loss of consciousness
- Coma
- Heart failure
- Death

Treatment

The treatment of electrolyte imbalances depends on what type of electrolyte is affected. For example, if serum sodium levels are low, the treatment would include restriction of fluids; if sodium levels are too high, fluids should be replaced slowly by way of an intravenous saline solution.

A patient with low potassium levels should be urged to watch his/her diet and take potassium supplements. If a patient's potassium levels are high, the treatment should include diuretics, intravenous insulin, and potassium-depleting sodium polystyrene sulfonate.

Chapter 4: Neurological, Multisystem, and Behavioral Disorders

NEUROLOGICAL SYSTEM DISORDERS

Cerebrovascular Malformations

Cerebrovascular malformations are abnormal formations of the blood vessels in the brain. Examples include arteriovenous malformations and aneurysms.

Signs and Symptoms

The symptoms and signs vary depending on the size and location of the malformation, but generally, the possible symptoms include:

- Enlarged blood vessels
- Stroke
- Seizures
- Headache
- Depression
- Anxiety
- Memory problems

With arteriovenous malformation, the arteries and veins of the brain are directly connected to each other without the normal capillaries between them. When they are located in the dura, which is the outer covering of the brain, they are referred to as dural arteriovenous malformations. When just one artery and vein are involved, it is called an arteriovenous fistula. Arteriovenous malformations occur most often at the junction of cerebral arteries of the frontal lobe, frontal-parietal region, lateral cerebellum, and occipital lobe. They can compress brain tissue and lead to seizures, ischemia, and cerebral hemorrhage.

Symptoms associated with dural arteriovenous malformations, in addition to those mentioned above, are difficulties with vision and hearing. Clients often complain about a pulsating sound inside their head.

Treatment

Superficial arteriovenous malformations less than 3 cm in diameter are typically corrected with a combination of radiosurgery, microsurgery, and endovascular surgery. Deep arteriovenous malformations less than 3 cm in diameter are treated with stereotactic radiosurgery, endovascular therapy, and coagulation with focused proton beams.

Aneurysms

An aneurysm of the brain, also known as a cerebral aneurysm, occurs from a weakness in the wall of the cerebral artery or vein. They are more commonly seen in adults rather than in children, and they usually result from a congenital connective tissue defect like pseudoxanthoma elasticum, Ehlers-Danlos syndrome, or autosomal dominant polycystic kidney syndrome or a pre-existing condition such as head trauma, atherosclerosis, or hypertensive vascular disease.

Cerebral aneurysms are usually small, less than 2.5 cm in diameter. They can be classified as saccular (noncircumferential) or as berry aneurysms, which have small, berry-like pouches. Most occur in the anterior and middle arteries or at the circle of Willis.

The Signs and Symptoms

The signs and symptoms that can be experienced prior to the rupture of an aneurysm include nausea; vomiting; loss of consciousness; severe headaches (thunderclap headaches), which can come on suddenly; eye pain; and diplopia and other impairments of vision including a complete visual loss. In some instances, there are no symptoms noticed at all.

Aneurysms are diagnosed with CT angiography, magnetic resonance angiography, and angiography.

Treatment

Because asymptomatic aneurysms in the anterior region of the brain less than 7 mm rarely rupture, no treatment may be necessary other than follow-up monitoring. Conversely, larger aneurysms of the posterior circulation can be life-threatening because of cerebral compression and hemorrhage. Endovascular surgery is needed.

ENCEPHALOPATHY

Encephalopathy refers to brain disease, damage, and malfunction. Encephalomyelopathy is a broadly used term, but most of the time, another word precedes it to describe the reason, cause, or condition the patient has that leads to the brain malfunction. For example, hepatic encephalopathy is a malfunction of the brain caused by liver disease, and metabolic encephalopathy is associated with metabolic disorders.

Signs and Symptoms

A commonly occurring symptom relating to all forms and types of encephalopathy is an altered state of consciousness. Other possible symptoms are:

- Tremors
- Seizures
- Dementia
- Lethargy
- Muscle twitching and myalgia
- Cheyne-stokes respirations
- Coma

The severity of the symptoms depends on the gravity of the brain disease and resulting damage.

Prevention

Encephalopathy can be prevented and limited when the underlying cause is identified and adequately treated. For example, hepatic encephalopathy can be avoided through the avoidance of alcohol intoxication, drug overdose, and injection of illegal intravenous drugs. Infectious encephalopathy can be prevented by avoiding contact with anyone possibly infected with organisms like N meningitis and shigella, which can cause encephalopathy.

Complications

The complications of encephalopathy depend on the type and severity of the encephalopathy. The complications can range from no or minor complications to severe complications that can lead to death.

Treatment

The treatment of encephalopathy is directly dependent on the cause. Treatments can vary greatly since the cause of the disease varies considerably. Some treatment options include oxygen therapy, rehabilitation, IV fluids, organ transplants, medications, etc.

INTRACRANIAL HEMORRHAGE

An intracranial hemorrhage is bleeding that occurs inside the cranium. This bleeding can result from a hemorrhagic stroke, leakage of blood from an aneurysm in the brain, closed head trauma, and other reasons.

Hemorrhagic Stroke

Hemorrhagic strokes account for about 20% of all strokes. They are most commonly caused by hypertension; however, other risk factors include:

- Vascular cerebral malformations
- Tumors
- Head trauma
- Ruptured aneurysms

Cerebral injury occurs as the result of decreased perfusion and increased intracranial pressure.

Subarachnoid Hemorrhage

A subarachnoid hemorrhage is when blood leaks into the subarachnoid space from a cerebral vessel. This is not a commonly occurring cause of a stroke, but it does sometimes happen. A subarachnoid hemorrhage is a serious medical emergency that results from a ruptured cerebral aneurysm, a spontaneous subarachnoid hemorrhage, or a severe closed head injury that occurs as the result of trauma. The prognosis for subarachnoid hemorrhage is poor.

People between the ages of 40 and 60 years are at greatest risk for a subarachnoid hemorrhage secondary to an aneurysm. Other risk factors include a family history of subarachnoid hemorrhage, cigarette smoking, and hypertension.

Symptoms and Signs

The symptoms and signs of subarachnoid hemorrhage occur most commonly during strenuous activity. The onset is sudden and unexpected. Many clients who present in the emergency department with complaints of a postcoital headache may have experienced a subarachnoid hemorrhage.

Other signs and symptoms include:

- Nausea and vomiting
- Upper neck pain and stiffness
- Slurred speech
- Extreme hypertension
- Decreased level of consciousness
- Mental changes such as depression, confusion, delirium, and apathy

Treatment

The ultimate goals of treatment include the prevention of bleeding and rebleeding, the maintenance of adequate oxygenation, and the reduction of both increased intracranial pressure and hypertension.

Other treatment options include:

- Anticonvulsant therapy to manage seizures
- Analgesics to ease pain and discomfort
- Antiemetic for vomiting
- Surgical clipping of aneurysms, if necessary
- Oral nimodipine to decrease the risk of vasospasm and cerebral ischemia

Epidural Hematoma

An epidural hematoma occurs when a blood clot, or hematoma, forms between the skull and the brain. Epidural hematomas primarily occur as the direct result of a traumatic head injury such as a severe fall or a serious blow to the head. An epidural hemorrhage is relatively easy to treat, and, in most cases, it has a good prognosis.

Signs and Symptoms

The signs and symptoms usually develop quite quickly. Some patients will lose consciousness briefly, and when they regain consciousness, they often insist they are asymptomatic. Others lose consciousness, and unfortunately, they will not regain consciousness, even with treatment. Many do not survive.

Treatment

The two treatment options are immediate surgery and initial conservative observation, which can lead to delayed evacuation. The underlying cause must also be addressed and treated. For example, traumatic increases in intracranial pressure must be decreased or reversed to keep the patient alive.

Encephalitis

Encephalitis is the swelling and inflammation of the brain as the result of an infection. When a pathogen causes inflammation of the patient's brain tissue, cerebral edema and destruction of nerve cells occur. This destruction of nerve cells causes intracerebral hemorrhage, increased intracranial pressure, and brain damage.

Signs and Symptoms

Mild cases of encephalitis can present with symptoms similar to those of a common cold such as mild fever, slight headache, fatigue, and loss of appetite.

Other symptoms can include:

- Drowsiness
- Confusion
- Disorientation
- Clumsiness and unsteady gait
- Stiff neck and back
- Nausea and vomiting
- Photosensitivity
- Irritability

Encephalitis in an infant or newborn is harder to diagnose, but some of the signs and symptoms are:

- Vomiting
- A fontanel, or soft spot on the head, may bulge
- Poor eating
- Excessive crying
- Body stiffness

Symptoms that signal a medical emergency include:

- Severe headache
- Seizures
- Muscle weakness or paralysis
- Loss of consciousness, poor responsiveness, stupor, coma
- Sudden mental function changes such as lack of effect, inappropriate mood, amnesia, poor decision-making, impaired judgment, and social withdrawal

Prevention

The prevention of encephalitis includes avoiding others with infectious diseases and avoiding contact with mosquitoes. This avoidance of mosquitoes can be achieved by applying insect repellent, removing standing water sources, and wearing clothing that covers as much of the body as possible.

The rabies virus can also cause encephalitis, so vaccination of pets is actively encouraged. Other preventive vaccinations available for humans include measles, herpes zoster, and viral encephalitis vaccinations.

Complications

A possible complication of encephalitis, in severe cases, is permanent brain damage that can affect the patient's hearing, memory, vision, speech, sensation, and muscular control.

Treatment

The ultimate goal of treatment for encephalitis is to ensure patient comfort, adequate fluid, adequate nutrition, and rest.

Medications used include:

- Antibiotics when bacteria cause the infection
- Acetaminophen for fever and headache
- Sedatives to treat restlessness and irritability
- Steroids to reduce cerebral swelling, like dexamethasone
- Antiseizure medications like phenytoin
- Antiviral medications to treat herpes encephalitis, for example acyclovir (Zovirax) and foscarnet (Foscavir)

Speech therapy and physical therapy may be necessary for those with severe, adverse effects from encephalitis.

SEIZURE DISORDERS

Abnormal electrical activity in the brain is the cause of seizures. Seizures can be an acute primary event or the result of a cerebral trauma or insult such as a stroke.

Energy and oxygen demand significantly increase during a seizure. Both cerebral energy demands and cerebral blood flow demands increase by 250% during a seizure, and cerebral oxygen demands increase by about 60%. Increased cerebral blood flow is the body's way of compensating for increased glucose and oxygen needs during a seizure.

Many clients experience an aura or partial seizure prior to a tonic-clonic seizure. They may also experience warning symptoms days or hours before the seizure.

Some of the risk factors associated with seizures include:

- Alzheimer's disease
- Alcohol withdrawal
- Some prescription medications
- Kidney or liver failure
- High blood pressure
- Hypoglycemia
- Toxin exposures
- Brain tumors
- Brain infection (previous or current)
- Use of illegal drugs or drug overdose
- Blood relatives with history of seizures
- Stress

- Flashing lights
- Some diseases such as sickle cell anemia, Whipple's disease, etc.
- Hormonal changes
- Syphilis

The Classification of Epileptic Seizures

The International Classification of Epileptic Seizures differentiates between partial and generalized seizures.

Partial seizures, also referred to as focal seizures, can be subcategorized as simple partial, complex partial, or secondary generalized seizures, as determined by the presence or absence of a loss of consciousness.

- A simple partial seizure involves no loss of consciousness. These seizures are characterized by somatic sensory symptoms (visual changes, auditory impairments, olfactory disturbances, and "pins and needles"), autonomic nervous system signs and symptoms (grimacing, chewing, lip-smacking, and picking at an object), focal-clonic motor signs and symptoms (Jacksonian March), and mental changes (feelings of déjà vu and jamais vu).

- A complex partial seizure leads to changes in the level of consciousness. The response to external stimuli is reduced with this type of seizure. Consciousness is lost when seizure activity spreads to the deeper portion of the brain and to another cerebral hemisphere.

When a patient is suffering from generalized seizures, his/her motor function is abnormal from the beginning, and usually, they become unconscious. Some of the subcategories of generalized seizures are:

- Infantile spasms
- Typical absence seizures
- Atypical absence seizures
- Atonic seizures
- Tonic seizures
- Tonic-clonic seizures
- Myoclonic seizures
- Juvenile myoclonic epilepsy
- Febrile seizures
- Status epilepticus

Infantile spasms present only during the first five years of life. They last only a few seconds, but can occur several times a day. Developmental defects are associated with these seizures.

Typical absence seizures are accompanied with a 10 to 30-second period of unconsciousness without convulsions. The patient has no recollection of these seizures. Typical absence seizures are most common among children who have genetically inherited this disorder. If there is no treatment given for these seizures, they can occur several times a day, and they often occur when the patient is simply sitting quietly. They do not typically occur in patients who are moving around or exercising. There is usually no sign in neurological and cognitive tests to diagnose these types of seizures.

Atypical absence seizures usually occur in patients with Lennox-Gastaut syndrome. This syndrome is a severe form of epilepsy. The onset of these seizures usually begins before the patient is four years old. They last longer than typical absence seizures, and the jerking movements that occur are usually more pronounced as well. These patients suffer a less severe loss of awareness than those with typical absence seizures. These seizures will often continue through adulthood. Patients who suffer from these types of seizures show abnormal results in their neurological tests and often have a history of developmental delays and some kind of nervous system damage.

Atonic seizures most often occur in children with Lennox-Gastaut syndrome. Children experiencing these types of seizures will fall to the ground, which puts them at risk of suffering head trauma. The patient will present with a short-lived complete loss of both muscle tone and consciousness.

Tonic seizures usually occur in children while they are asleep. The cause of these seizures is usually Lennox-Gastaut syndrome. This type of seizures lasts about 10-15 seconds each.

Tonic-clonic seizures can appear in different ways. They can be primarily or secondarily generalized. In the primarily generalized form of these seizures, the patient cries out and then falls and loses consciousness. The muscles of the extremities, trunk, and head will then rapidly begin contracting and relaxing. There is also the occasional occurrence of tongue biting, frothing of the mouth, and urinary and fecal incontinence. The seizure lasts one to two minutes. The secondarily generalized form of these seizures starts with a simple partial or complex partial seizure.

Myoclonic seizures are short-lived seizures. Single limbs, several limbs, or the trunk can experience quick jerking motions during these seizures. They are not accompanied by loss of consciousness unless they turn into generalized tonic-clonic seizures, which is sometimes the case.

Juvenile myoclonic epilepsy is an epilepsy syndrome that normally presents in adolescents. Patients with this form of epilepsy suffer from myoclonic, tonic-clonic, and absence seizures. These seizures present in the morning after the patient has not slept well or has consumed alcohol.

Febrile seizures occur in patients with a fever, but who are not suffering from an intracranial infection. They are considered a provoked type of seizure. Three to five percent of children between the ages of three months and five years are affected by these types of seizures. There are two types of these seizures: benign and complicated. In the benign form of these seizures, the patient experiences a short, solitary, and generalized seizure that is tonic-clonic in appearance. The complicated form of these seizures can last more than 15 minutes and can recur two or more times during a 24-hour period.

Status epilepticus is a life-threatening condition. Under this condition, a patient's brain is in a state of persistent seizure. It is one continuous seizure that lasts for over five minutes or several seizures in which consciousness is not regained between seizures, which last for over five minutes each. Patients suffering from these types of seizures should always be considered as going through a medical emergency and thus treated that way.

Generalized seizures are also subcategorized as generalized tonic-clonic seizures and non-convulsive seizures.

- Generalized tonic-clonic seizures, previously known as grand mal seizures, are marked with a sudden loss of consciousness; stiffening and extension of arms and legs; forceful jaw closure; a shrill cry or noise; urinary and/or fecal incontinence; tachycardia; profuse diaphoresis; increased salivation; hyperventilation; eye-rolling; cyanosis; pupil dilation; apnea; and a lack of papillary responses to light rhythmic, alternating periods of muscular contraction and muscular relaxation.

  After the seizure, the client may be confused, fatigued, irritable, and complain of a headache and muscular pain. People who have experienced this type of seizure have no memory of it.

- Nonconvulsive seizures, which are also referred to as absence seizures, mostly affect children from 4 years of age to puberty. These seizures typically last only a few seconds and do not induce muscular relaxations and contractions. Some of the signs and symptoms of this type of seizure include eye-rolling; twitching or drooped lips; a blank, trance-like stare; and a lack of responsiveness to verbal stimuli.

The client is assessed for the presence of any seizure risk factors. An electroencephalogram (EEG) is completed to record and evaluate brain waves and to rule out epilepsy as the cause of the seizure activity. An MRI and CT scan are completed to determine if there are any brain abnormalities such as a cerebral tumor. A lumbar puncture is completed to determine whether or not the client has an infection or bleeding. A magnetocnccphalography (MEG) is completed to assess, and PET imaging is completed to ascertain the location of the seizure activity.

Signs and Symptoms

Most seizures are short-lived and last less than a couple of minutes. It is a life-threatening medical emergency when the seizure lasts more than five minutes, when the client does not return to a normal level of consciousness, and when the client experiences several seizures in succession.

Treatment

The ultimate goal of treatment is to address and remove the cause of the seizure. Some of the treatments include medications like Ativan, Cerebyx, Dilantin, luminal, Depakote, and Topamax; sometimes, surgery is indicated. For example, a client may undergo a surgical procedure to remove a small area of the brain that is causing the seizures. Additionally, the client should be taught to understand the warning signs of a seizure, to avoid factors that place him/her at risk for them, and to wear a medical emergency tag or bracelet that alerts others to his/her seizure disorder.

CEREBROVASCULAR ACCIDENTS (STROKE)

Strokes are a major neurological event that can lead to permanent disability and death.

Symptoms and Signs

The symptoms and signs of stroke vary according to the type of stroke and the area of the brain adversely affected by the stroke. The anterior circulation oxygenates and nourishes the retina, temporal lobe, frontoparietal lobe, and optic nerve. The signs and symptoms affecting this area include dysphagia, visual alterations, sensory and motor facial deficits, mathematical and writing difficulties, motor and sensory deficits affecting a leg, urinary deficits, personality changes, and unilateral neglect that typically affects the left side.

Conversely, the posterior circulation supplies the temporal lobe, occipital lobe, brain stem, thalamus, and cerebellum. The signs and symptoms, therefore, include vertigo, nystagmus, and ataxia that are related to cerebral deficits; visual disturbances; bilateral or unilateral sensory and motor deficits; vertigo; and diplopia.

Strokes affecting the brainstem typically present with altered levels of consciousness and loss of other functions associated with the brainstem.

Strokes are classified according to the cause of the stroke.

Ischemic Stroke

Simply stated, ischemic strokes deprive the brain of its essential blood and oxygen supply. These strokes result from three major pathological processes including emboli, thrombi, and hypoperfusion.

Embolic strokes occur when a blood vessel is occluded by a clot that can originate from some different places including the major vessels of the heart and the legs. The risk factors are atrial fibrillation and valve disease, although some can be caused by a fat embolus, a septic embolus, or the result of illicit intravenous drug abuse.

Thrombosis, or the narrowing of blood vessels, secondary to clot formation is one of the most common causes of a stroke. Risk factors for this type of ischemic stroke include atherosclerosis, some infectious diseases, and vasculitis. Thrombolytic medications should be administered within three to four and a half hours after the onset of symptoms.

Hypoperfusion is a rare type of stroke and can occur as the result of a cardiac dysrhythmia.

Treatment

Aspirin, if given within 48 hours of the onset of symptoms, is beneficial to reducing mortality and recurrent stroke. Prior to this administration, intracerebral hemorrhage should definitively be ruled out with a CT. The use of other anticoagulants, like low-molecular-weight heparin, is not recommended for ischemic stroke patients. Anticonvulsant drugs, like phenytoin, treat seizures that can often occur after an ischemic stroke.

Hemorrhagic Stroke

Cerebral injury occurs as a result of decreased perfusion and increased intracranial pressure. Hemorrhagic strokes are most commonly caused by hypertension, but other causes like those below can also lead to this kind of stroke:

- Vascular malformations
- Tumors
- Head trauma
- Hemorrhage caused by a ruptured aneurysm

Treatment

Intracerebral hemorrhage management depends on the cause, location, client clinical condition, and any neurological deficits. Cerebral edema and increased intracranial pressure must be carefully monitored.

Transient Ischemic Attacks

Transient ischemic attacks (TIA) closely mimic stroke with the exception that transient ischemic attacks cause temporary neurological deficits that last only a short period and without permanent disability. Despite their quick resolution, however, transient ischemic attacks are a serious warning sign of impending stroke.

Treatment

The primary focus of immediate care is the identification and treatment of the cause. Supplemental oxygen is used to maintain cerebral perfusion. Antiplatelet medications liked ticlopidine, aspirin-dipyridamole, and clopidogrel help prevent other TIAs and stroke. Other interventions aim to decrease the client's risk factors. For example, a preventive carotid endarterectomy may be indicated for those at risk for clots. Additionally, diabetes, hypertension, and hyperlipidemia must be controlled to decrease the client's risk.

MULTISYSTEM DISORDERS

PRESSURE ULCERS

Pressure ulcers, also known as bedsores, pressure sores, and decubiti, are injuries that occur as a result of excessive pressure on the skin. They can affect both the surface of the skin and the tissues that surround the area. Pressure ulcers are most common on bony areas (such as ankles, heel, hips, or buttocks) that are subjected to pressure and among the cognitively impaired, elderly, clients with neurological impairments, incontinent patients, and those who are immobile.

Immobile patients and those unable to move around freely are at a higher risk than are mobile patients because excessive and constant pressure on one spot results in a pressure ulcer. Each position in bed, like the supine and lateral side-lying positions, has its unique pressure points, as listed below:

- Prone position: Knees, toes, genitalia, breasts, shoulder, cheek, and ear
- Supine position: Sacrum, heels, elbows, scapulae, and back of head
- Lateral position: Shoulder, ileum, ear, greater trochanter, knee, and ankle
- Fowler's or sitting position: Pelvis, sacrum, vertebrae, and heels of feet

There are four stages, based on severity, in which pressure ulcers fall. As defined by the National Pressure Ulcer Advisory Panel, these stages are:

- **Stage I**

  The following characteristics are experienced at the beginning stage of a pressure sore:

  o The skin remains unbroken and intact.
  o There is either no color change, a blue-purple hue, or an ashen appearance among those with darker skin; on people with a lighter skin color, the skin appears reddened among people with lighter skin color.
  o The skin does not blanch.
  o Site itchiness
  o Site may be soft, firm, painful, and either cooler or warmer than the surrounding skin.

- **Stage II**

  This is a partial thickness wound of the epidermis, dermis, or both. Stage II pressure ulcers are open wounds. The skin is not intact.

  - o The pressure ulcer appears as a shallow, basin-like wound, pinkish-red; a blister; a superficial abrasion; or a fluid-filled blister.
  - o There is damage on the part of the underlying dermis and epidermis.

- **Stage III**

  The ulcer is a deep, full thickness wound with some necrosis and undermining damage that extends beyond the visible surface wound. It consists of all levels of the skin and the subcutaneous tissue to the fascia.

  - o The loss of the epidermis and dermis expose fat tissue.
  - o The damage may extend below layers of healthy skin beyond the primary wound.
  - o A yellowish necrotic tissue, called slough, may be in the deepest portion of the wound.
  - o The ulcer looks like a crater.

- **Stage IV**

  A stage IV ulcer includes large-scale loss of tissue including destruction of underlying muscles, supporting fascia, tendons, and possible bone and joint capsule involvement. Sinus tracts are common, and the deepest portion of the wound may have slough as well as eschar.

Prevention

Prevention of pressure sores requires repositioning at least every two hours, or more often as indicated. Other preventive measures include good skin care, regular skin assessments, good nutrition, gel cushions, use of repositioning devices, special supportive mattresses, maintenance of clean and dry skin despite incontinence, and prevention of friction and shearing when the patient is being positioned and repositioned.

The skin should be cleansed with a mild moisturizing soap and then dried completely with a soft towel. Bland, non-scented lotion should then be applied to keep the skin soft and pliable. Bowel and bladder schedules should be consistent in order to prevent moisture, which contributes to skin breakdown. Incontinence products, like briefs, are not a substitute for toileting and good skin care.

A nutritious diet can decrease risk. The diet should include ample amounts of fiber, fluids, vitamins, and minerals. Supplemental iron; vitamins A, C, and B complex; and selenium, copper, zinc, and manganese are often used. Additionally, 1 ½ to 2 daily grams of protein and additional calories should be provided according to the patient's albumin levels. A high protein, high calorie diet is needed to treat malnutrition.

Special pressure-reducing devices should be a part of standard care. High-risk patients should have a flotation mattress or an alternating pressure mattress; activity, ambulation, or position changes should be provided at least every two hours.

All patients should be screened for pressure ulcer risk. When a patient is identified as at risk for pressure ulcers, special preventive measures should immediately be implemented.

Complications

Some of the complications of pressure ulcers include sepsis, bone and joint infections, pain, increased lengths of stay, and increased healthcare costs.

Treatment

The goals of wound care for pressure ulcers include cleaning and debriding the wound, covering and protecting the wound, treating any local infection, and supporting wound healing.

Sterile normal saline is used to clean the wound. This cleansing is followed by loosely filling the wound with wet saline-fluffed gauze to fill the dead space and then covering the area with a wet-to-moist dressing.

A debriding agent can be applied or surgical debridement can be performed when indicated. Cultures will be needed when cellulitis is present.

Local antibiotic ointments can also be prescribed. Wound and dressing coverings are specific to the status of the wound. Their purpose is to speed the migration of fibroblasts and epithelial cells to the surface of the wound edges to begin the healing by secondary intention.

Other interventions include pressure relief, a nutritious diet, and pain management.

Dressing	Mechanism of Action	Stage 1	Stage 2	Stage 3	Stage 4

Dry gauze	Wicks drainage away from wound surface			X	X
Wet-to-damp gauze	Maintains moist wound environment; wicks drainage away from wound surface			X	X
Transparent barrier	Retains wound moisture; allows gas exchange; does not stick to wound surface	X	X		
Hydrocolloid	Occlusive; repels moisture and dirt; maintains moist wound environment	X		X	
Hydrogel	Maintains moist wound environment		X	X	X
Alginate	Maintains moist wound environment; absorbs exudate			X	X

Kozier, Barbara, Glenora Erb, Audrey Berman, and Shirlee Snyder. Fundamentals of Nursing: Concepts, Process, and Practice. 7th ed., pp. 873, "Table 34-5." Prentice-Hall, 2004.

NOSOCOMIAL HEALTHCARE-ACQUIRED INFECTIONS

Most nosocomial infections are spread by the hands of healthcare workers from one patient to another. These infections are limited to only those that a patient did not have before he/she was hospitalized or cared for, but acquired after admission or after care was provided.

The most commonly occurring risk factors for nosocomial infections are prolonged illness and immunosuppression, which can result from an infection like HIV; treatments such as chemotherapy; and some medications. Additionally, all pieces of equipment and nonsterile supplies can harbor and spread nosocomial infections. Nosocomial infections are quite costly and they can, for the most part, be prevented.

The urinary tract, respiratory tract, wounds, and bloodstream are the most common sites for nosocomial infections; some of the commonly occurring pathogens include E.coli, candida albicans, staphylococcus aureus, pseudomonas aeruginosa, and enterococcus.

Hand washing is the single most effective way to prevent nosocomial infections in healthcare facilities. Protective precautions such as standard precautions and transmission-based precautions are also necessary to prevent the spread of these deadly infections; prevention is extremely important because of the presence of so many resistant strains of pathogens like methicillin-resistant staphylococcus penicillin-resistant streptococcus pneumoniae, vancomycin-resistant enterococcus (VRE), and aureas (MRSA).

Protective precautions include:

- Standard precautions that apply to all blood and bodily fluids and all clients, regardless of the person's diagnosis

- Contact precautions to prevent direct and indirect contact transmissions, as those contained in diarrhea, wounds, and herpes simplex

- Airborne precautions for the prevention of airborne transmission microbes like TB. These precautions include a HEPA mask and a negative pressure room.

- Droplet precautions to prevent the transmission of pathogens that are transmitted with a cough or sneeze. Masks are indicated for these precautions.

Infections Transmitted With Blood and Other Bodily Fluids

Some of the infections and diseases transmitted via blood and bodily fluids are:

- HIV
- Hepatitis type B
- Hepatitis type C
- Herpes simplex and other sexually transmitted infections

HIV/AIDS

The etiology of human immunodeficiency virus (HIV) is caused by the HIV-1 and HIV-2 retroviruses that deplete helper T-4 cells. This compromises cellular immunity.

The risk factors include:

- IV drug use using contaminated needles
- Unprotected sex, multiple sexual partners, genital lesions, and anal sex
- Perinatal exposure during pregnancy

These infections can range from primary asymptomatic infection to overt AIDS, which is often complicated with opportunistic infections that can lead to death. Opportunistic infections can affect the pulmonary system, nervous system, and musculoskeletal system.

Some opportunistic infections include:

- Pneumocystis carinii pneumonia
- Kaposi's sarcoma
- Candidiasis
- Cytomegalovirus

- Herpes simplex
- Histoplasmosis
- Mycobacterium avium infection
- Salmonella
- Toxoplasma gondii
- Tuberculosis

Other complications include acid-base imbalances, fluid and electrolyte disorders, blindness, and peripheral neuropathy.

Signs and Symptoms

Fever, malaise, dyspnea, lethargy, skin rash, chills, night sweats, dry cough, oral lesions, diarrhea, weight loss, abdominal discomfort, headaches, stiff neck, confusion, lymphadenopathy, progressive edema, and seizures are some of the signs and symptoms associated with HIV/AIDS.

Treatment

HIV/AIDS is treated with highly active antiretroviral therapy (HAART). The goals of this treatment are to decrease the viral load, to prevent secondary infections, to increase the CD4 T cells, and to maintain the client in the best possible level of health. Compliance and patient education is critical to the success of this treatment because these medications must be taken for life.

The medications in a HAART regimen are classified as:

- Protease inhibitors (lopinavir/ritonavir)
- Fusion inhibitors
- Nucleoside reverse transcriptase inhibitors (zidovudine)
- Nonnucleoside reverse transcriptase inhibitors (Efavirenz)
- Combination antiretroviral agents (Combivir and Trizivir)

Hepatitis Type B and Hepatitis Type C

Viral hepatitis is a major liver infection. It has three phases:

- Preicteric Phase:
  Fatigue, nausea, joint pain, anorexia, and cough may be present. Laboratory values reveal elevated ALT and AST with elevated urine bilirubin levels.

- Icteric Phase:
  This phase is characterized with dark urine, clay-colored stools, jaundice, right upper abdominal quadrant pain, pruritis, and elevated direct bilirubin levels.

- Posticteric Phase:

Laboratory values approach normal levels, but malaise and fatigue may continue. There is decreasing jaundice, an improvement of appetite, and lightening of urine with stool returning to normal color.

Treatment

Generally, all medications except those absolutely necessary are avoided because the liver metabolizes medications. Chronic hepatitis C is treated with interferon; at times, vitamin K may be needed for prolonged prothrombin times.

Sexually Transmitted Diseases

Sexually transmitted infections and diseases are transmitted through sexual contact, but some, like syphilis, can be contracted by the fetus in utero.

The tables on pages 92-93 list some known sexually transmitted diseases and their associated causative agents, infectious agent types, incubation periods, signs and symptoms, and treatments.

	Syphilis	**Gonorrhea**	**Chlamydia**
Causative Agent	Treponema pallidum	Neisseria gonorrhea	Chlamydia trachomatis
Type of Infectious Agent	Bacteria	Bacteria	Bacteria
Incubation Period	Usually 3 weeks, with a range from 9 days to 3 months	Men: 3-30 days Women: 3 days to an indefinite number of days	
Signs and Symptoms	Primary: chancres Secondary: fever, weight loss, jaundice, rash, patchy alopecia	Men: urethritis; dysuria; burning; frequency; white, yellow, or green penis discharge; and painful, swollen testicles	No signs at times. Possible Signs: Female: vaginal discharge,

	Latent: no signs Late: tumor-like mass (gumma), meningitis, paralysis, lack of coordination, paresis, confusion, delusions, impaired judgment, slurred speech, and tabes dorsalis	Women: yellow or blood vaginal discharge, dysuria, frequency, burning, feeling of fullness or discomfort in abdomen/pelvis, vaginal bleeding with intercourse	burning with urination, irritation, bleeding after sexual intercourse, lower abdominal pain Male: urethritis
Treatment	Penicillin G	Ciprofloxacin	Azithromycin or doxycycline

	Trichomoniasis	**Genital/ Oral Herpes**	**Human Papillomavirus**
Causative Agent	Trichomonas vaginalis	Herpes simplex	Condylomata acuminata
Type of Infectious Agent	Protozoa	Virus	Virus
Incubation Period		3-7 days	

Signs and Symptoms		Vague nonspecific signs like vaginal or urethral discomfort and others such as generalized signs of infection, local inflammation, pain, and lesion on the vagina or external genitalia of males	
Treatment		Antiviral medications: acyclovir, famciclovir, and valacyclovir	

Compiled by the author (Monahan, F. D. et al. <u>Phipps Medical-Surgical Nursing: Health and Illness Perspectives</u>. 8th ed, p 1336, "Table 46-5". Mosby, 2007.)

URINARY TRACT INFECTIONS (UTIs)

E. coli is the offending pathogen associated with urinary tract infections among females. Females are at greater risk for UTIs than males because of their anatomical differences in terms of a shorter urethra and the structural proximity of the urethra to the rectum, vaginal canal, and coital secretions. Klebsiella, proteus, and staphylococcus, in addition to E.coli, can also cause urinary tract infections. Males typically present with a urinary tract infection secondary to some obstructive process.

The client assessment will reveal dysuria; frequency; urgency; nocturia; pain and discomfort in the suprapubic area; and hematuria, gross or microscopic, with the presence of a urinary tract infection.

Nursing interventions include:

- Encouraging a daily fluid intake of 2500-3000 ml (3 liters)
- Administering antibiotics

- Instructing the client regarding:

  o Avoiding bladder irritants such as caffeine, alcohol, cola drinks, and asparatame
  o Voiding as soon as possible after coitus
  o Avoiding external irritants such as bubble baths, perfumed vaginal cleansers or deodorants, and talcum powder
  o Hygiene (washing the perineal area while standing in the shower, not in the tub)
  o Wiping front to back after each void and bowel activity
  o Wearing cotton panties only
  o Changing sanitary pads at least every three hours

CATHETER AND CENTRAL LINE-ASSOCIATED INFECTIONS

Catheter-associated urinary tract infections (CAUTI) and central-line-associated blood steam infections (CLABSI) are major concerns in healthcare. All invasive procedures and treatments such as these place patients at risk for infection.

Catheter-Associated Urinary Tract Infections (CAUTI)

Urinary tract infections can affect any area of the urinary system including kidney, ureters, bladder, and urethra. Urinary tract infections are the most frequently occurring nosocomial, or healthcare-associated, infections, and the vast majority of these cases are associated with a urinary catheter, particularly when the catheter is in place for an extended period of time.

Preventive measures of catheter-associated urinary tract infections include:

- Inserting and using urinary catheters only when necessary
- Removing the catheter as soon as possible
- Inserting, caring, and maintaining the catheter only by those competent to do so
- Maintaining strict aseptic technique
- Using sterile supplies and equipment
- Maintaining unobstructed urinary flow
- Hand washing
- Maintaining a closed urinary drainage system without disconnecting the catheter from the tubing or the tubing from the drainage bag
- Always keeping the catheter and bag lower than the level of the bladder to prevent urinary backflow
- Avoiding any kinking or twisting of the catheter
- Securing the catheter to the leg to avoid catheter pulling
- Emptying the collection bag frequently and not touching the drainage spout with anything

Some alternatives, like a portable ultrasound device to assess urine volume and silver-alloy coated catheters and other antimicrobial-impregnated catheters may also reduce catheter-associated urinary tract infection risks by eliminating the need for catheterization and preventing infection, respectively. Additionally, external condom catheters should be considered for male patients, and intermittent catheterization, rather than an indwelling catheter, should also be considered.

Some of the common symptoms of a urinary tract infection are:

- Lower abdominal pain or burning
- Fever
- Hematuria, which can indicate a urinary tract infection or another disorder of the urinary tract
- Burning during urination
- Urinary frequency and urgency

PALLIATIVE CARE

Palliative care, also referred to as comfort care, is in contrast to curative care. Palliative care supports the client and family at the end of life rather than continuing to treat the cancer. Many clients who choose palliative care choose to cease all medications and treatments other than those that relieve the symptoms at the end of life. It aims to improve the patient's quality of life, taking into account his/her emotional, physical, and spiritual needs as well as the needs of loved ones.

Palliative care can be provided at any time throughout a serious illness or disease. Palliative care helps to relieve pain or other symptoms the patient may have and helps the patient and loved ones to completely understand the condition and how to cope with it.

END OF LIFE

There are some cases in which a patient has a life-threatening incurable disease or disorder. The physician can give him/her options of procedures or treatments that can be given in which there is a possibility that the patient's life can be extended. In some of these cases, the patient may choose to stop treatment, which can mean dying sooner, but maybe more comfortably. The patient may want to establish advance directives, which can allow loved ones and healthcare providers to know exactly what the patient's wishes are, and these patients may choose to plan their funeral.

At the end of life, comfort care measures are available to make the patient more comfortable and to ease their symptoms. Medication is also still available for these patients to assist with pain or discomfort from their illness. Some patients may choose to die peacefully at home, whereas others may choose to enter a hospital or hospice.

Comfort Care Measures

There are several different measures aside from medications that can be used for relief from pain and/or a variety of other symptoms. Some measures can be more helpful to one patient, where others may be more helpful to others. There are some patients who even use a combination of measures to achieve the relief they need.

These comfort care measures include:

Massage

Massage decreases stress and pain. Relaxation techniques, soothing music, and soft lighting, combined with massage, is a great way to help alleviate stress and pain to promote sleep, rest, and circulation. It also conveys caring and compassion as part of the nurse-client relationship, and it also gives the nurse a chance to speak with the client about his/her concerns.

Massage can include hand massage, back massage, foot soaking and massage, and neck massage. A warm lotion or oil is used for the massage.

Meditation

Meditation is thought to reduce fatigue, stress, and anxiety, all of which are often experienced by oncology clients. During meditation, the client should be instructed to concentrate on his/her breathing while repeating positive and calming phrases in his/her mind. Meditation is spiritual; prayer is often religious.

Prayer

Prayer is a helpful method for a cancer patient, survivor, and loved ones. These prayers can be religious in nature or non-religious. They can be composed of specific prayers associated with a certain religion or prayers that are in one's own words.

Heat and Cold Applications

Heat and cold applications can be quite helpful in the reduction of pain, but as with any other treatment, it is necessary to consult the treating physician before administering. The heat can be helpful in reducing the pain associated with sore muscles. It can be applied with a heating pad, gel packet, warm water bottle, or hot bath or shower. Heat should not be used for more than 10 minutes at a time.

Cold can help relieve or ease pain in a patient by numbing it for a period of time. Cold can be administered by cold gel packs, frozen peas, or ice cubes wrapped in a cloth. As with hot treatments, cold treatments should be used for a maximum of 10 minutes.

Deep Breathing

Deep-breathing techniques are used by cancer patients, and are shown to be effective for tension, anxiety, and fatigue.

Progressive Muscular Relaxation

Progressive muscular relaxation (PMR) therapy aims to reduce the feeling of tension, to lower perceived stress, and to induce relaxation in the patient. It involves progressively tensing and releasing major skeletal muscle groups. Its goals are to reduce the stimulation of the autonomic and central nervous system and to increase parasympathetic activity.

It has been reported that patients who use progressive muscular relaxation experience a reduction in their state of anxiety, pain, and symptoms of depression. It also improves sleeping habits and overall quality of life.

Distraction

According to the American Cancer Society, distraction means turning your attention to something other than the pain. Distraction aims to manage mild pain or, with medications, to deal with severe pain. While waiting for pain medication to start working, distraction is quite helpful. Some forms of distraction are watching television, talking on the telephone, and other things that can help patients take their mind off the pain they are experiencing.

Imagery

The American Cancer Society explains imagery, which is also referred to as guided imagery or visualization, as mental exercises intended to aid the mind's influence over the well-being and health of the body. The patient creates a kind of purposeful daydream by imagining sights, smells, tastes, and other pleasant sensations.

Imagery is helpful in reducing stress, anxiety, and depression; managing pain; lowering blood pressure; and easing some of the side effects of chemotherapy. Overall, imagery aims to create a general feeling of being in control.

Biofeedback

Biofeedback is a method of treatment in which the patient is able to use monitoring devices to help consciously control physical processes that are normally controlled automatically; temperature, heart rate, sweating, blood pressure, muscle tension, and sweating, for example.

It has been shown that biofeedback can help patients with chronic pain and sleeping difficulties, and it can help improve the patient's overall quality of life.

Hypnosis

Self-hypnosis and hypnosis produces a state that includes relaxation and deep concentration. It is helpful for reducing pain, fear, anxiety, and fatigue among oncology clients.

Transcutaneous Nerve Stimulation (TENS)

A transcutaneous nerve stimulator, also referred to as a TENS unit, is used as a method of pain relief by transmitting low-voltage electrical impulses through electrodes placed on the skin on or around where the pain is.

This device can provide the patient with short-term pain relief, but it has not been shown to provide long-term relief.

Acupuncture

This ancient Chinese medical treatment uses very thin needles, which are placed in the skin, and helps reduce pain, nausea, and vomiting.

Acupressure

Acupressure is similar to acupuncture, but it uses pressure instead of needles. It can be quite helpful for nausea.

Mind-Body Exercises

Mind-body exercises combine deep-focused breathing, movement, and meditation. These exercises can help the oncology client combat stress, depression, and fatigue. Yoga and tai chi are two examples of mind-body exercises.

Herbs

Herbs and dietary supplements are helpful for many oncology patients. Some herbs reduce vomiting and nausea; others help decrease pain and fatigue. For example, astragalus, which comes from the astragalus plant's root, can boost the immune system. Vitamins like vitamins A, C, E, and coenzyme Q 10 may provide some protection against cancer, but it is not substantiated in professional literature.

HOSPICE

Hospice care is an option for patients with serious diseases and disorders who feel that the treatments they have received and are currently receiving are not benefiting them.

Patients can be admitted to hospice to receive assessment and pain relief, as well as care for other distressing signs and symptoms they are dealing with.

The ultimate goal of hospice care is to provide patients with expert care in a calm and soothing environment that makes the client feel at home and comfortable. Hospice care treats all patients with the utmost care and dignity to ensure their comfort and the comfort of their loved ones.

INFECTIOUS DISEASES

Organisms such as bacteria, viruses, fungi, and parasites cause infectious diseases. Infectious diseases are passed in different ways. For example, some are passed from person-to-person, some are passed through the ingestion of contaminated foods, and others are acquired by getting bitten by an insect or animal.

There are a variety of different signs and symptoms that each type of infectious disease carries, although the most common are chills and fever. These diseases and their symptoms can vary so greatly that some patients require only home remedies to get better, whereas others are so serious that they can be life-threatening and can require hospitalization. Influenza is a common infectious disease, and some more serious infections are multi-drug resistant organisms such as MRSA and VRE.

The Chain of Infection

There are five aspects of the chain of infection: the causative agent, reservoir, portal of exit, mode of transmission, and portal of entry.

- The Causative Agent:
  The offending pathogen can be bacteria, virus, fungus, rickettsial organism, protozoa, or helminth (worm).

- The Reservoir:
  The reservoir is the place in which the pathogen lives and grows. Reservoirs can include animal, human, and inanimate (soil, water/fluid, equipment) places. When the pathogen normally lives, and thrives, in the mucous membranes or skin of the host, it is called an endogenous reservoir; all other reservoirs are exogenous sources.

- The Portal of Exit:
  The portal of exit is the pathway where the agent leaves the reservoir. Portals of exit can be the respiratory tract, GI tract, genitourinary tract, open lesions on the skin, and across the placenta.

- The Mode of Transmission:
  The agent needs a mode of transportation to enter a new host. This transmission mode, or method of transportation, can be through the air, with direct contact,

or via a vehicle or vector. Contact transmission includes direct, indirect, and droplet contact.

- The Portal of Entry:
  The pathogen or causative agent's entry portals are similar to the exit portals, and they can include the respiratory, gastrointestinal, and genitourinary systems in addition to any opening in the skin, mucous membranes, and across the placenta.

- The Susceptible Host:
  The susceptible host is a person who is susceptible to the infection. For example, people with weakened immune systems are more susceptible to infectious agents than those with intact immune systems.

Any break in the chain of infection will prevent infection.

Modes of Transmission

- Droplet transmission occurs when the agent leaves the reservoir in droplets such as occurs with a sneeze or cough.

- Airborne transmission differs from droplet transmission because the agent remains suspended in the air as a droplet nuclei or dust. The susceptible host inhales the pathogen with air flow.

- Direct contact occurs with direct physical contact or skin shedding into the susceptible host.

- Indirect contact occurs when there is an intermediate, inanimate object between the source of infection and the susceptible host. This inanimate object, called a fomite, may be bed linen, respiratory equipment, a door handle, a toothbrush, or silverware.

- Common vehicle transmission is described as when an inanimate object, or fomite, serves as an intermediary for an infection of multiple susceptible hosts. For example, salmonellosis-contaminated water, air, food, and fluids and hepatitis A are examples of common vehicle transmission microorganisms.

- Vector-borne transmission occurs when an animate, living thing, other than a human, carries the infectious agent from one host to another. For example, Lyme disease is carried by a tick, and Rocky Mountain spotted fever is carried by a mosquito.

91

The Stages of Infection

The stages of infection are:

- The Incubation Period:
  The incubation period is the amount of time after entry that the pathogen spreads through the body.

- The Prodromal Stage:
  The prodromal stage is marked with signs and symptoms including fever, sore throat, etc. The person is contagious in this stage and can spread the infection to others.

- The Acute Stage:
  The acute stage consists of the period of maximum illness. Local or systemic infection is occurring.

- The Convalescence Stage:
  The infection resolves during this stage. Convalescence can take days or even months, depending on the infection and the severity of it.

There are numerous types of infectious agents including:

- Bacteria
- Viruses
- Fungi
- Prions

MULTIDRUG-RESISTANT ORGANISMS

Multidrug-resistant organisms are bacteria that have become resistant to medications, usually an antibiotic, used for treatment. Bacterial infections are treated with antibiotics. When one antibiotic fails to effectively treat the infection, the infection is called drug-resistant, and the organism is referred to as resistant or multi-resistant.

Multidrug-resistant organisms are most often found in a hospital or long-term care facility. They cause severe infections, such as MRSA or VRE, and usually affect the elderly and the severely ill more often than others.

METHICILLIN-RESISTANT STAPHYLOCOCCUS AUREAS (MRSA)

Methicillin-resistant Staphylococcus aureus (MRSA) infection is a strain of the staphylococcus bacteria that has become resistant to the antibiotics usually used to treat them.

Healthcare-associated MRSA (HC-MRSA) is nosocomial MRSA, which occurs at a healthcare facility or hospital. Community-associated MRSA (CA-MRSA) is the type of MRSA contracted by people out in the community.

It usually starts out as a painful skin boil that can be transmitted through contact with the skin. It is often found among child-care workers, high school wrestlers, and other people who live in crowded conditions.

Signs and Symptoms

MRSA usually begins as small red pimple or boil-like bump. Quickly, these little bumps turn into deep, very painful abscesses, which must be surgically drained. In some occasions, the bacteria burrows deeply into the body, which can then cause potentially life-threatening infections located in the joints, bloodstream, heart valves, lungs, surgical wounds, and bones.

It is not uncommon for MRSA to lead to sepsis and death.

Prevention

Hospital-based MRSA is prevented by:

- Standard precautions
- Isolation
- Use of personal protective equipment like gowns, gloves, masks, and goggles
- Strict hygiene
- Scrupulous hand washing
- Sterilization
- Disinfection

Community-based MRSA is prevented by:

- Good hygiene including hand washing and disinfection
- Keeping wounds covered
- Avoiding sharing of personal items such as towels, sheets, razors, clothing, and other contaminated items
- Showering immediately after athletics
- Sanitizing linens if a cut or sore is present. All laundry should be washed and dried on the hottest settings.

Complications

MRSA infections are able to resist common antibiotics, thus making them difficult to treat. When untreated, it will spread to other parts of the body such as the bloodstream, joints, bones, lungs, and heart, therefore become life-threatening.

Treatment

HC-MRSA and CA-MRSA may be able to be treated with an effective antibiotic. In some instances, the use of antibiotics may not even be necessary. For example, a superficial abscess caused by MRSA can be drained rather than attempting to treat the infection with an antibiotic.

VANCOMYCIN-RESISTANT ENTEROCOCCI (VRE)

When a sensitive enterococcus cell acquires a special piece of DNA, called plasmid, vancomycin resistance occurs. This new enterococcus strain is called vancomycin-resistant enterococci (VRE).

VRE organisms are usually resistant to more than one antibiotic, and it is spread from person-to-person.

Symptoms and Signs

Depending on the site of the infection, different symptoms may present. For example:

- VRE in the bloodstream is sepsis, which leads to symptoms that can include fever, tachycardia, malaise, and weakness.

- Urinary tract infections cause symptoms such as back pain, fever, and burning while urinating.

- Meningitis, which is uncommon, can cause symptoms such as headache, stiff neck, confusion, and fever.

- Heart valve infection, which is endocarditis, causes prolonged sepsis and can cause a leak or failure of the valve.

- Pneumonia can cause coughing, difficulty breathing, shortness of breath, respiratory compromise, and fever.

Prevention

Preventing the transmission is the best way of preventing the cause. Hospitals and long-term care facilities should adhere to infection control guidelines. Other tips include washing hands before and after using the restroom and washing up before and after touching the mouth and nose. IV catheters and urinary catheters should be avoided whenever possible, and antibiotics should be used only when appropriate. For example, antibiotics should not be used to treat viruses like the common cold.

Treatment

Most microbiological laboratories can supply the treating physician with a combination of newer and older antibiotics that can treat the VRE. If they cannot, the state lab or the CDC should be contacted. They should be able to help. If there is a collection of pus, such as an abscess, it is important that it be drained.

PAIN

Pain is covered above under End of Life Care.

THE SEPSIS CONTINUUM

Sepsis continuum is a continuum of clinical manifestations from systemic inflammatory response (SIRS) to sepsis to severe sepsis to septic shock. It includes the full range of responses from SIRS to organ dysfunction to multiple organ failure and ultimately, death.

SIRS

Systemic inflammatory response syndrome results from an infection. Having two or more of the following symptoms can be indicative of SIRS:

- Abnormal white blood cell count
- Fever of more than 100.4° F
- Greater than 20 breaths per minute respiratory rate
- Greater than 90 bpm heart rate

SIRS is not always caused by an infection; in some instances, it can be caused by inflammation, trauma, ischemia, or a combination of these things.

Sepsis

Sepsis can be uncomplicated in nature, such as when caused by viral infections like the flu, gastroenteritis, or dental abscesses. This form of sepsis is very common and in the majority of cases, no hospitalization is required.

Severe Sepsis

When sepsis occurs and there is a problem in one or more of the patient's vital organs such as the lungs, heart, kidneys, or liver, it is known as severe sepsis. Patients with severe sepsis are more likely to be very sick and at a greater risk of death than those with uncomplicated sepsis.

Septic Shock

Septic shock occurs when a patient suffers from sepsis and has low blood pressure. The usual treatment of fluid administration and use of vasopressors does not work, which leads to problems in one or more of the vital organs, as discussed in the severe sepsis section above. Patients with severe sepsis are extremely ill and do not get enough oxygen for their body to function properly. This condition is considered a medical emergency requiring immediate intensive care unit admission. Even with the best treatment, the death rate for patients with septic shock is about 50%.

SHOCK STATES

Shock is the state in which the body tissue is unable to properly perfuse because the body's demand for nutrients and oxygen exceeds the available amount.

Hypovolemic Shock

Hypovolemic shock is the most common type of shock. Primarily, hypovolemic shock results from hemorrhage or the loss of fluid from the body's circulatory system. Patients at risk of this type of shock are those who suffer from burns, extreme dehydration, diabetic ketoacidosis, and diabetes insipidus and those who have been exposed to environmental hazards.

The signs and symptoms that a patient may experience as a result of hypovolemic shock include pale skin; oral dryness; poor skin turgor; and excessive thirst, which is a sign of dehydration being present. Due to diminished circulating hemoglobin, tachypnea can occur.

The four stages or classifications associated with hypovolemic shock can range from stage one in which patients exhibit minimal clinical signs and a minimal amount of fluid loss to stage four in which over 40% of the total volume of fluid is lost. Often, this stage is irreversible and can be life-threatening to the patient.

Anaphylactic Shock

Anaphylactic shock typically occurs as the result of an allergic response to a medication such as penicillin; another common reason is an extreme allergic reaction to a type of food or a bite from a bee or wasp. The immune system causes a gross relaxation of the blood vessels. Histamine is released, as well as other vasodilator substances, which relaxes most of the vascular smooth muscle. The patient's blood pressure drops, and there is pooling of venous blood, which impairs the blood's return to the heart and cardiac output.

Edema occurs in the laryngeal mucosa caused by the antigen-antibody reaction. An allergic rash and bounding heart may also be present. Rapid death can occur. Anaphylaxis is a life-threatening sensitivity reaction.

If the cause of the anaphylaxis is an IV antibiotic to which the patient is allergic, the IV must be removed immediately. Adrenaline or noradrenaline is also given immediately in order to reduce laryngeal edema and to constrict the vasculature.

BEHAVIORAL DISORDERS

ALTERED MENTAL STATUS AND LEVELS OF CONSCIOUSNESS

An altered mental status is defined as a change in awareness of a person's surroundings and/or impaired mental functioning. There are many causes for an altered mental status, and some examples are infections, an adverse drug reaction, hypoxia, electrolyte imbalances, very high or very low blood glucose levels, delirium, and dementia.

Altered mental status can range from minor confusion to coma, and it is associated with safety risks. Mental status is a combination of a patient's level of consciousness and his/her level of cognition.

A complete history should be obtained including a determination of:

- Any prior history of changes in the level of consciousness
- Any traumas like a fall or assault
- The time of the change in the level of consciousness
- Any signs and symptoms like infection, etc.
- Any drug or alcohol abuse or use
- Any environmental factors including exposure to carbon monoxide, etc.

The physical assessment relating to altered levels of consciousness includes:

- An assessment of priority issues like increased intracranial pressure, hypoxia, and easily treatable hypoglycemia

- A neurological exam and vital signs. Hypothermia can be the cause of the altered consciousness, and hyperthermia can indicate an infectious cause of altered levels of consciousness.

- The assessment of the pupils for size, reactivity to light and accommodation, and equality as part of the neurological assessment. Pupil dilation is an indication of increased intracranial pressure.

The Glasgow Coma Scales for adults and children are standardized assessment tools for altered levels of consciousness.

Signs and Symptoms

The signs and symptoms associated with an altered mental status include excessive sleepiness, strange behavior, altered thinking, difficulties with concentration, and decreased arousal senses.

Treatment

In order to treat an altered mental status, the first step is to make sure that vital body functions are supported, which can include intravenous fluids and oxygen therapy.

It is vital that all patients with an altered mental status are protected at all times from self-harm.

DELIRIUM

Delirium is a serious disturbance to a patient's mental abilities. The patient will suffer a decreased awareness of his/her surroundings and confusion. Delirium comes on suddenly, usually within a few hours or over a few days, and it can, in most cases, occur as the result of one or more of the following:

- Severe or chronic mental illness
- Medications
- Infections
- Surgery
- Drug or alcohol abuse

Signs and Symptoms

There are several signs and symptoms of delirium. It is important to note that patients with delirium often times experience bouts of delirium interspersed with periods of lucidity. This can make it more difficult to diagnose.

The primary symptoms of delirium include:

- Reduced awareness of the environment, which can include an inability to stay focused on one topic or an inability to change topics, wandering attention, being withdrawn with no response to the environment, easily distracted by unimportant things, and getting stuck on one idea instead of being able to answer simple questions.

- Cognitive impairment, which can present as difficulty reading, writing or understanding speech; disorientation; inability to recognize people, places, or things; rambling in nonsensical speech; problems speaking or understanding words; and poor short-term memory.

- Behavioral changes such as extreme emotions like fear, anxiety, depression, or anger; changes in sleep habits; restlessness; agitation; irritability; combative behavior; and hallucinations.

Prevention

The only prevention for delirium is to avoid the risk factors that can cause an episode to occur. For hospitalized patients, these risk factors can include loud noises, poor lighting, a lack of natural light, invasive procedures, and frequent room changes. There are certain things the hospital staff can do to prevent an episode of delirium from being triggered. These include providing:

- Pain management
- Natural forms of sleep and anxiety management
- Noise reduction
- Prevention of sleep interruptions
- Mobility and range of motion exercises
- Stimulating and familiar activities
- Adequate fluids
- Comfortable communication

Complications

The length of delirium can last anywhere from hours to several months, and if the factors that contributed to the delirium are addressed, the recovery time is decreased. When the patient's level of health prior to the delirium is good, he/she is likely to recover fully.

Delirium among the seriously ill can result in permanent thinking and/or functioning level disabilities. The seriously ill can also have a general decline in their overall health and need for institutionalization, poor recovery after surgeries, and a risk for mortality.

Treatment

Treatment for delirium requires immediate discontinuation of the cause or trigger of the delirium. Once that has been addressed, it is then necessary to create an optimal environment in which the patient can recover.

Supportive care should be given to the patient in order to prevent complications from occurring. This includes protecting the airway; providing the patient with sufficient fluid and nutrition; assisting them with movements, as needed; providing pain management; and keeping the environment familiar and the patient oriented.

Avoiding medications that trigger delirium is also essential. Some medications can be helpful for treating symptoms like hallucination, severe agitation, confusion, fear, and paranoia.

DEMENTIA

Dementia is not considered a specific disease, but rather a group of symptoms that affect a patient's thinking and social abilities so severely that they interfere with the patient's everyday life and functioning. Unlike delirium, which can be treated and reversed, most cases of dementia are not reversible.

A patient with dementia has a problem with two or more brain functions, which include memory loss; impaired judgment or language; and inability to perform typical daily functions such as bill paying, grocery shopping, laundry, etc.

Alzheimer's syndrome is the number one cause of progressive dementia.

Signs and Symptoms

The signs and symptoms of dementia vary depending on the actual cause of the dementia. Signs and symptoms include:

- Hallucination
- Memory loss
- Agitation
- Paranoia
- Personality changes
- Problems performing usual activities

Prevention

The exact prevention of dementia is not known, but it has been shown that the following does help:

- Keeping an active mind
- Staying active, both physically and socially
- Ceasing smoking
- Lowering blood pressure to a normal level
- Eating healthful

Complications

Complications associated with dementia can include:

- Communication problems
- Emotional health deterioration
- Sleeping difficulties
- Reduced hygiene
- Delusions and hallucinations

- Inadequate nutrition
- Forgetting to take medications

Treatment

The majority of dementia types cannot be cured. Treatment involves management of symptoms, which can help slow or minimize the development of additional symptoms. Some helpful medications include memantine and cholinesterase inhibitors.

Chapter 5: Psychological Disorders

The commonly occurring signs and symptoms of mental illness are not as clear and objective as the signs and symptoms of a physiological disorder. Generally, the signs and symptoms of mental disorders can include abnormal changes in mood, social withdrawal, changes in thought processes, changes in personal habits, and other behaviors.

THE CLASSIFICATION OF MENTAL ILLNESSES

The most commonly occurring mental illnesses are:

- Substance abuse disorders such as alcohol abuse or drug dependence
- Personality disorders such as dependent personality and antisocial personality
- Eating disorders
- Anxiety disorders such as obsessive disorders, phobias, and panic disorders
- Mood disorders such as bi-polar and depression
- Sleep disorders
- Schizophrenia and other psychotic disorders such as paranoid or catatonic-type schizophrenia
- Sexual and gender identity disorders
- Cognitive disorders such as dementia and delirium
- Impulse control disorders

The American Psychiatric Association's Diagnostic and Statistical Manual of Mental Disorders (DSM) contains four major categories of mental illnesses. Each of these categories contains hundreds of related mental health disorders and their characteristics. These categories are:

- Behavioral disorders
- Mood disorders
- Thought disorders
- Mixed disorders

Mental illness can also be categorized, or classified, as temporary, episodic, or chronic. Bi-polar disease and schizophrenia, for example, are considered episodic mental illnesses because the client has periods of lucidity interspersed with the symptoms of the mental illness. Examples of chronic and permanent mental illnesses are irreversible dementia and non-relenting bi-polar disease and schizophrenia.

ANXIETY DISORDERS

Anxiety disorders are marked with characteristic physiological symptoms and responses. Some of the most commonly occurring anxiety disorders are:

- Generalized anxiety disorders
- Obsessive compulsive disorders
- Panic disorders
- Phobias

Anxiety disorders can completely consume the client and make him/her unable to enjoy and/or participate in the activities of normal living. These disorders can occur as the result of a combination of stressful life events and personality traits like excessive worrying and ungrounded, irrational fears.

The Signs and Symptoms of Anxiety Disorders

Mild Anxiety

Anxiety can be classified as mild, moderate, severe, and panic level. Some of the signs and symptoms of mild anxiety include:

- Mild agitation
- Restlessness
- Tension-diffusing behaviors like fidgeting
- Irritability
- Attention-seeking behaviors
- Mild, slight discomfort and uneasiness

Moderate Anxiety

The signs of moderate anxiety are:

- Shaking
- Memory alterations
- Poor concentration
- Decreased attention span
- Voice tremors
- Tachypnea
- Tachycardia
- Increased muscular tension and aches
- Pacing and other forms of extreme tension

Severe Anxiety

The signs of severe anxiety are:

- Tachycardia
- Hypertension
- Shortness of breath and other respiratory symptoms
- Hyperventilation

- Rapid speech
- Feeling of impending doom and dread
- Confusion
- Somatic complaints
- Dizziness, nausea, vomiting, headache, and sleeplessness

Panic Level Anxiety

The signs and symptoms associated with panic level anxiety are:

- Pupil dilation
- Severe dizziness
- Immobility
- Feelings of absolute terror and fear
- Severe hyperactivity and possible exhaustion
- Tremors
- Chest pain
- Heart palpitations
- Inability to communicate with others
- Hallucinations
- Delusions

Because some of these symptoms mimic life-threatening physical disorders such as an airway obstruction or an impending myocardial infarction, physiological disorders are ruled out before a psychological disorder, such as an anxiety disorder, is diagnosed.

Treatment

Minor tranquilizers such as clorazepate, diazepam, and lorazepam are used to control, but not cure, overwhelming anxiety. Other treatment strategies include:

- Identifying and assessing the client's coping mechanisms
- Facilitating the client to develop more effective and appropriate coping mechanisms
- Encouraging the client to verbalize beliefs about the stressors in his/her life
- Encouraging the client to effectively cope with the present stressors in his/her life
- Discussing, and teaching the client, the ways he/she can better resolve conflicts

Treatment after discharge is typically done in the community with a combination of medications, cognitive behavioral therapy, and community support or recovery programs under the direction of the client's psychiatric care team.

DEPRESSION AND SUICIDE

Patients suffering from depression and/or who have attempted suicide previously are at greatest risk for suicide.

The Signs and Symptoms of Severe Depression and Suicide Risk

- Expressions of helplessness and/or hopelessness
- Notes or words that say "goodbye"
- A sense of guilt and/or shame
- Changes in eating, appetite, and/or sleeping patterns
- Severe drop in school or work performance
- Dramatic changes in personality or appearance
- Irrational, bizarre behavior
- A lack of interest and enthusiasm about the future
- Giving away personal possessions
- Self-harming actions like a drug overdose or a failed hanging

The Assessment of the Suicidal Client

All healthcare personnel should always approach the patient with empathy and care for his/her well-being. The ultimate goal of treatment is to prevent suicide and return the client to the community when he/she is safe.

As the client is being assessed, the nurse should conversationally focus on:

- The degree of suicide intent
- The client's suicide plan
- The duration of the depression
- Any precipitating factors that led to the depression
- The client's current feelings about death

Treatment

The priority treatment consists of measures to relieve the depression, to prevent suicide, and to preserve life. This treatment includes a combination of medications and ongoing cognitive behavioral therapy.

Some of the medications for depressed clients include antidepressants, antipsychotic medications, and antianxiety agents. Antidepressants are the most commonly prescribed medications for patients with depression.

SUBSTANCE ABUSE

Substance abuse is the dependence on or overindulgence in an addictive substance, such as illegal drugs and/or alcohol. As with the abuse of some types of illegal drugs, alcohol withdrawal occurs when a chronic user of alcohol suddenly stops drinking.

Chronic Alcohol Abuse

Chronic alcohol abuse is drinking on a regular basis to the point of intoxication or drinking to the level of intoxication in a sporadic manner. Chronic alcohol abuse can cause many serious medical, psychological, social, and occupational problems. Chronic alcohol abusers often hurt their loved ones, and they cause serious emotional, financial, and physical damage to the family unit and friends.

Alcohol Withdrawal

Alcohol withdrawal can lead to a variety of symptoms when a chronic alcohol abuser suddenly discontinues drinking.

Symptoms of withdrawal can range from mild to severe, and they can also be physical and/or psychological. Some examples of mild to moderate psychological symptoms are shakiness, nervousness, anxiety, depression, fatigue, and bad dreams. Mild to moderate physical symptoms include sweating, headache, nausea and vomiting, pale and clammy skin, tachycardia, and tremors. Severe physical symptoms include agitation, fever, convulsions, and a confused state known as delirium tremens. These severe symptoms can lead to injury and even death.

The treatment for alcohol withdrawal depends on several factors including severity of dependence, length of dependence, client age, and client health.

Chronic Drug Abuse

Chronic drug abuse is defined as the habitual abuse of legal prescription drugs and/or illicit drugs to the extent that the abuse significantly injures the user with physical, social, or economic harm.

Drug-Seeking Behavior

Drug-seeking behavior is a pattern of behavior with which a person tries to obtain prescription medications such as narcotic painkillers, anxiety medication, and tranquilizers using a variety of illegal strategies and mechanisms including:
- False identification
- Forged or adjusted prescriptions
- Repeated requests for refills for "lost" or "stolen" medication
- Falsely reporting pain or anxiety
- Abusive or threatening behavior when denied medications

Chapter 6: Professional Caring and Ethical Practice

According to the American Association of Critical Care Nurses (AACN), nursing care is the integration of the knowledge, experience, skills, and abilities to care for patients and families using eight primary competencies as discussed below. All eight of these competencies are essential for quality care, but each one can become a priority, as based on the client's characteristics. Synergy results when these competencies are aligned with client needs; the whole becomes greater than the sum of the parts.

Clinical Judgment: According to the American Association of Critical Care Nurses, "clinical reasoning including clinical decision-making, critical thinking, and a global grasp of the situation, coupled with nursing skills acquired through a process of integrating education, experiential knowledge, and evidence-based guidelines."

All nurses must be critical thinkers. Patient care and patient needs are much more complex and multivariate than in the past. A great deal of uncertainty, ambiguity, and vagueness challenge the nurse, particularly in progressive care. Situations are not always straightforward and clear. Critical thinking combines problem-solving, decision-making and creative skills. Traits that characterize critical thinkers are confidence, courage, tolerance for ambiguity, perseverance, curiosity, autonomy, intellectual expertise, high levels of motivation, and open-mindedness.

All interventions should be based on the nurse's experiential knowledge, education, and best practices and evidence-based practices. Using evidence-based practices is a highly beneficial method to determine the best implementation strategies. Evidence-based practice is research-based practice. These practices can, and should, be accessed using a wide variety of current professional journals and databases.

Advocacy/Moral Agency: According to the American Association of Critical Care Nurses, "working on another's behalf and representing the concerns of the patient/family and nursing staff; serving as a moral agent in identifying and helping to resolve ethical and clinical concerns within and outside the clinical setting."

Nurses serve as an advocate for the client when they defend client rights to quality care, when they uphold client rights and dignity including the right to autonomous decision-making, and when they morally and ethically resolve concerns and possible ethical dilemmas.

The American Nurses Association's Code of Ethics applies to all nurses in all settings and in all specialty practices including progressive care. This code emphasizes the dignity and worth of all people without discrimination, nurses' commitment to patients, advocacy, accountability, the preservation of safety and patient rights, competency, the provision of quality care, collaboration, and the integrity of the nursing profession.

Ethical principles include:

- Autonomy and Self-Determination: Each unique individual has the right to make choices without coercion or the undue influence of others. Progressive care nurses do not impose their own beliefs, values, or opinions on the client. They accept all client choices without any judgments. The patient has the right to choose and/or refuse any and all treatments and interventions.

- Non-maleficence: Non-maleficence means "do not harm," as in the Hippocratic Oath. Harm can be intentional or unintentional, as is the case when a client has an adverse reaction to a medication.

- Beneficence: Although beneficence may appear to be the opposite of non-maleficence, it is not. Beneficence simply means "do good." Doing good is more than just not doing any harm (non-maleficence). On occasions, beneficence can lead to unanticipated harm.

- Justice: The principle of justice requires nurses to be fair to all. For example, limited resources must be fairly and justly distributed among all patients.

- Fidelity: Fidelity is being faithful to one's promises. By the very nature of the implicit nurse-client relationship, the nurse must be faithful and true to his/her professional promises and responsibilities by providing high-quality, safe care in a competent, scientifically grounded manner.

- Veracity: Veracity is truthfulness. Nurses do not withhold the whole truth from clients.

- Accountability: Nurses are accountable for all aspects of nursing care. They must answer to themselves, their clients, and society at large for their actions. They must also accept personal and professional consequences for all of their actions.

Caring Practices: According to the American Association of Critical Care Nurses, "nursing activities that create a compassionate, supportive, and therapeutic environment for patients and staff with the aim of promoting comfort and healing and preventing unnecessary suffering. These caring behaviors include, but are not limited to, vigilance, engagement, and responsiveness of caregivers. Caregivers include family and healthcare personnel."

Caring involves complete connectedness with the client. The nurse skillfully and intentionally connects to the client to transmit feelings of emotional and physical security. Caring actively involves the client in a mutual relationship of trust and recognition.

Collaboration: According to the American Association of Critical Care Nurses, "Working with others (e.g. patients, families, and healthcare providers) in a way that promotes/encourages each person's contributions toward achieving optimal/realistic patient/family goals. Collaboration involves intra- and interdisciplinary work with colleagues and the community."

Nurses communicate and collaborate with virtually all other members of the healthcare team including those in the community. The client is the center of care, and therefore, all nurses also actively collaborate with the client and family members relating to all aspects of care and treatment. Some of the skills needed for collaboration include communication and decision-making skills and the ability to establish and maintain mutual trust and respect.

Systems-Thinking: According to the American Association of Critical Care Nurses, "Body of knowledge and tools that allow the nurse to manage whatever environmental and system resources that exist for the patient/family and staff within or across healthcare systems and non-healthcare systems."

Systems, including humans, are a set of interacting, identifiable parts or components that continuously interact with others and the environment through input, throughput, output, and feedback, which goes into the system as input. Negative feedback inhibits change, and positive feedback stimulates change. Systems-thinking facilitates holistic care and a view of multidimensional human beings in constant interaction with others and the environment.

Systems theory, as put forward by Bertalanffy, states that all systems are self-regulating because they can correct themselves as the result of feedback. According to this non-particulate theory, the whole (the human being) is greater than the sum of its particulates, or parts.

Response to Diversity: According to the American Association of Critical Care Nurses, "The sensitivity to recognize, appreciate, and incorporate differences into the provision of care. Differences may include, but are not limited to, individuality, culture, spirituality, gender, race, ethnicity, lifestyle, socioeconomics, age, and values."

Although the terms *culture* and *ethnicity* are used synonymously, they are not. Culture is a set of practices, customs, beliefs, and attitudes passed from generation to generation and not shared by others outside of the culture. An ethnic group shares a common characteristic such as a language, and race is based on a physical or genetic trait like skin color. The U.S. is often referred to as a "melting pot" of many diverse cultures and people of virtually all ethnicities. Nurses and other healthcare providers must incorporate patients' specific cultural and ethnical needs into all aspects of care.

Madeleine Leininger put forth the Theory of Transcultural Nursing, also referred to as the Culture Care Diversity and Universality Theory, to provide nurses with a better and fuller understanding of culture and the effect of culture on the client and his/her needs.

During the assessment phase of the nursing process, the nurse assesses the client's and family members' cultural background, preferences, and needs. After this assessment is complete, the nurse can generate a plan of care that addresses these critical factors. This cultural assessment and culturally oriented care enables the nurse to discover ways that the client's culture and faith systems impact his/her experiences with illness, suffering, and even death. It also helps nurses to:

- Integrate cultural knowledge into the treatment of patients. This open-mindedness may lead to non-traditional, alternative nursing interventions such as spiritually based therapies like meditation and anointing.

- Remain fully respectful of human diversity

- Strengthen their commitment to culturally based nurse-patient relationships, which emphasize the importance of the whole person rather than the patient as simply a set of symptoms or an illness.

Leininger states that caring is the unifying, universal, dominant, and distinctive essence of nursing. Caring is culturally driven, as based on the rich tapestry of variations among cultures' patterns, processes, and expressions. Madeleine Leininger supports three nursing modes of intervention necessary to care for, and assist, people of diverse cultures. These three nursing modes are:

- Cultural care accommodation and negotiation, or both
- Cultural care restructuring and repatterning
- Cultural preservation and maintenance

Culture is integral to the person as a unique individual. It greatly impacts the client's health and his/her reactions to treatments and care.

Facilitation of Learning: According to the American Association of Critical Care Nurses, "The ability to facilitate learning for patients/families, nursing staff, other members of the healthcare team, and the community. This includes both formal and informal facilitation of learning."

The phases of the teaching/learning process are the same as the phases of the nursing process: assessment, diagnosis, planning, implementation, and evaluation.

The purpose of assessment is to determine the client's learning needs; level of motivation and readiness; personal, ethnical, and cultural aspects; age-specific characteristics and needs; and barriers to learning including cognitive impairments, language, level of comprehension or reading level, and physical and psychological barriers to learning. Simply stated, a learning need equals what should be known minus what is actually known.

The diagnosis phase includes the generation of a nursing diagnosis based on analyzed assessment data. This diagnosis can include statements like "A lack of knowledge about…" and "A knowledge deficit related to…"

The purpose of planning is to ensure that patient/family teaching is consistent with identified learning needs and can be evaluated in terms of effectiveness (outcome evaluation). Planning consists of generating objective and specific learning goals, among other things. Learning objectives are specific, measurable, behavioral, learner-centered, consistent with assessed need, and congruent with the domain of learning. Examples of well-worded learning objectives are: "Patient will be able to list basic food groups" (cognitive domain) and "Patient will demonstrate coughing and deep-breathing techniques" (psychomotor domain).

The implementation phase consists of conducting the education activity in an environment conducive to learning that includes a physically comfortable environment, as well as one that is trusting, open, respectful, and accepting.

There are two types of evaluation in the teaching/learning process: formative and summative. Formative evaluation is the continuous assessment of the effectiveness of the teaching while the teaching is being conducted. It enables the teacher to modify the plan, if needed. Summative evaluation occurs at the end of the learning activity and allows the nurse to determine whether or not the education achieved the established learning objectives for the individual or group.

Some unique characteristics of learners include individual literacy, health literacy (the ability to understand information and use it to make appropriate healthcare decisions), learning style and preferences, cultural impacts on learning (communication patterns, vocabulary, slang, and/or terminology vary among and within many cultures), level of motivation/readiness, and presence of language barriers.

Clients will not learn unless they are motivated and ready to do so. Levels of motivation are assessed, and then the nurse aims to motivate the client with strategies such as focusing the learning on the solution of the client's current priority problems, involving the client in the entire teaching/learning process, and explaining the benefits of the learning in terms of the client's problem-solving and decision-making.

Language barriers can be overcome with techniques such as ongoing clarification and reclarification, speaking slowly, using diagrams, using pictures, and using the services of an interpreter. Cognitive limitations can be overcome with simple, slow, brief, and understandable explanations using aids such as pictures and diagrams. Additionally, learning can be facilitated for the visually impaired through the use of eyeglasses, Braille, magnifiers, and large-print reading material. Hearing-impaired clients benefit from hearing aids and a loud, crisp speaking voice directed toward them. Many can successfully lip-read.

Moderate stress motivates learning, but pain and severe stress impair learning. Nurses should establish trust to reduce stress and should address pain prior to a teaching/learning activity.

Clinical Inquiry: According to the American Association of Critical Care Nurses, "The ongoing process of questioning and evaluating practice and providing informed practice. This creates changes through evidence-based practice, research utilization, and experiential knowledge."

New knowledge is exploding as a result of the proliferation of scientific advances and research. It is difficult to remain current with this rapidly accelerating body of knowledge; however, despite the challenges, it is the responsibility of all nurses to remain current and competent in all these new areas.

It is also important for nurses to contribute to nursing's body of knowledge by participating in research. All nurses can, and should, participate in at least some aspects of the research process. Research is one of the provisions in the American Nurses Association's Standards of Practice for all registered nurses.

Evidence-based practice (EBP) is an approach to care that encourages clinicians to use in clinical practice the best available evidence, or research, in combination with the individual patient's circumstances and preferences. Simply stated, evidence-based practice is research-based practice.

Evidence-based practice begins with research. It is then developed into evidence-based nursing guidelines, which are disseminated through a wide variety of mechanisms including publication and professional conference. Lastly, it is used in practice. Some of the medical and nursing databases that nurses regularly use to review research and evidence-based practice are:

- The Cochrane Library
  http://www.thecochranelibrary.com/view/0/AboutTheCochraneLibrary.html

- The Joanna Briggs Institute
  http://www.joannabriggs.edu.au/

- Ovid's Evidence-Based Medicine Reviews (EBMR)
  http://www.ovid.com/webapp/wcs/stores/servlet/product_EvidenceBased-Medicine-Reviews-EBMR_13051_-1_13151_Prod-904

- Elsevier
  http://www.elsevier.com/

- Medlars
  http://www.nlm.nih.gov/bsd/mmshome.html

- Medline Plus (an international nursing index; IndexMedicus is also included)
  http://www.nlm.nih.gov/medlineplus/

- Pub Med
  http://www.ncbi.nlm.nih.gov/pubmed/

- The Cumulative Index to Nursing and Allied Health Literature (CINAHL)
  http://www.ebscohost.com/cinahl/

- The Directory of Open Access Journals
  http://www.doaj.org

- The Nursing Center for Lippincott Williams & Wilkins
  http://nursingcenter.com

Test Your Knowledge

1. Which serum biomarker confirms the presence of myocardial damage?
    A. Serum troponin
    B. Creatine kinase
    C. Myoglobin
    D. Antithrombin III

2. ST segment depression is a sign of:
    A. Ischemia, which may resolve with increased perfusion.
    B. Ischemia, which does not resolve with increased perfusion.
    C. Ischemia progressing to infarction.
    D. Ischemia with a high probability of infarction.

3. Which cardiac biomarker peaks 4-6 hours after an acute myocardial infarction?
    A. Creatine kinase
    B. Troponin T
    C. Troponin I
    D. Myoglobin

4. Thrombolytic therapy is indicated within how many hours after the onset of myocardial infarction symptoms?
    A. Less than 5 hours
    B. Less than 6 hours
    C. Less than 8 hours
    D. Less than 12 hours

5. Which cholesterol-lowering drug is associated with the side effect of gallstones?
    A. Niacin
    B. Gemfibrozil
    C. Ezetemibe
    D. Simvastatine

6. Which dietary recommendation is appropriate for the client with coronary artery disease?
    A. Monosaturated fats of < 10% of total calories
    B. Polysaturated fats < 20% of total calories
    C. Cholesterol < 200 mg/day
    D. Cholesterol < 300 mg/day

7. Sublingual nitroglycerine:
    A. May lead to a headache lasting up to about 20 minutes after administration.
    B. Can be taken up to two times in 10-minute increments before calling 911.
    C. Can be taken up to three times in five-minute increments before calling 911.
    D. Should be discarded after the original bottle has been opened for four months.

8. The PQRST mnemonic represents:
    A. What provokes or palliates the pain; Q represents the presence of a Q wave; R is any radiation to other areas of the body like the left arm or jaw; S is the severity of the pain; and T is the time and duration of the chest pain.
    B. What provokes or palliates the pain; Q represents the quality of the pain; R is any radiation to other areas of the body like the left arm or jaw; S is the severity of the pain; and T is an ST elevation
    C. What provokes or palliates the pain; Q represents the quality of the pain; R is any radiation to other areas of the body like the left arm or jaw; S is the severity of the pain; and T is the time and duration of the chest pain.
    D. What provokes or palliates the pain; Q represents the quality of the pain; R is any radiation to other areas of the body like the left arm or jaw; S is the severity of the pain; and T is the time and duration of the chest pain.

9. A clinical manifestation of cardiogenic shock is:
    A. A diastolic blood pressure of < 70 mmHg.
    B. A systolic blood pressure < 90 mmHg.
    C. A pulse rate of > 90 per minute.
    D. Increased left arterial pressure.

10. Sick sinus syndrome is associated with:
    A. Sinus bradycardia.
    B. Sinus tachycardia.
    C. Sinus arrest.
    D. Sinus tachycardia and bradycardia.

11. A risk factor associated with infective endocarditis is:
    A. Calcific aortic stenosis.
    B. Calcific mitral stenosis.
    C. Aortic valve prolapse.
    D. Pulmonary valve prolapse.

12. Which of the following statements is accurate relating to cardiac tamponade?
    A. It is a complication of endocarditis.
    B. It is a complication of myocarditis.
    C. It prevents the ventricles from filling.
    D. It prevents the atrium from filling.
13. Hypertensive crisis is manifested with:

A. A diastolic blood pressure above 100 mmHg and central nervous system compromise.

B. A diastolic blood pressure above 110 mmHg and central nervous system compromise.

C. A diastolic blood pressure above 120 mmHg and central nervous system compromise.

D. A diastolic blood pressure above 130 mmHg and central nervous system compromise.

14. Select the type of aortic aneurysm that is paired with its correct description.
    A. Fusiform aneurysm: The intimal layer of the aorta is affected.
    B. Fusiform aneurysm: The aneurysm radiates around the entire diameter of the aorta.
    C. Sacculated aneurysm: The aneurysm radiates around the entire circumference of the aorta.
    D. Pseudoaneurysm: The aneurysm involves only one side of the ascending aorta.

15. During the first stage of cardiogenic shock:
    A. The level of CO in the blood rises.
    B. Arterial blood pressure increases.
    C. Alkalosis occurs.
    D. Acidosis occurs.

16. An example of a stress-induced cardiomyopathy is:
    A. Takotsubo cardiomyopathy.
    B. Tokamu cardiomyopathy.
    C. Brugada syndrome.
    D. Brigada syndrome.

17. Takotsubo cardiomyopathy is characterized by:
    A. Possible reversal.
    B. Permanent cardiac damage.
    C. Male gender as a risk factor.
    D. Epicardial coronary artery disease.

18. Torsades de pointes is:
    A. An impulse conduction dysrhythmia.
    B. A bradydysrhythmia.
    C. A ventricular dysrhythmia.
    D. A device-related dysrhythmia.

19. A risk factor associated with first-degree AV block is:

A. An electrolyte balance.
B. Digitalis toxicity.
C. Hypertension.
D. Rheumatic fever.

20. Mobitz I is characterized by:
    A. Random non-conducted p waves.
    B. Patterns of non-conducted p waves.
    C. Constant P-R intervals.
    D. A widened QRS.

21. Select the type of edema that is paired with its correct description.
    A. 1+: 4 mm deep and barely visible.
    B. 2+: 4 mm deep and barely visible.
    C. 3+: 6 mm deep and rebounds in 10-20 seconds.
    D. 4+: 6 mm deep and rebounds in 10-20 seconds.

22. Ebstein's anomaly is:
    A. A congenital septal defect often seen in combination with an atrial septal defect.
    B. An acquired septal defect that can occur as the result of rheumatic fever.
    C. Associated with digitalis toxicity as a risk factor.
    D. Associated with heart failure as a risk factor.

23. The primary risk factor associated with a pulmonary embolus is:
    A. Immobility.
    B. Pneumonia.
    C. Deep-vein thrombosis.
    D. Peripheral vascular disease.

24. Prophylactic antibiotics are used with dental cleaning when the client is affected with:
    A. Mitral valve prolapse.
    B. Pericarditis.
    C. Rheumatic fever.
    D. Atrial septal defect.

25. Acute respiratory distress syndrome (ARDS):
    A. Can occur as the result of direct or indirect lung injuries.
    B. Is typically treated with CPAP therapy.
    C. Is typically treated with BPAP therapy.
    D. Occurs as the result of chronic obstructive pulmonary disease.

26. Select the phase of acute respiratory distress syndrome (ARDS) and its correct description.

A. Phase I: Intrapulmonary shunting, metabolic acidosis, and respiratory acidosis.

B. Phase II: Acute respiratory failure begins and diffuse rales occur.

C. Phase III: Acute respiratory failure begins and diffuse rales occur.

D. Phase IV: Respiratory alkalosis and metabolic alkalosis.

27. One of the presenting signs of chronic obstructive lung disease is:
    A. Slow, deep respiratory rate.
    B. Pain in the substernal area.
    C. A dry hacking cough.
    D. A cough with tenacious sputum.

28. Which adventitious breath sound is paired with its correct description?
    A. Pleural friction rub: A high-pitched sound
    B. Rhonchi: A low-pitched sound
    C. Pleural friction rub: A low-pitched sound
    D. Rhonchi: A high-pitched sound

29. Obstructive sleep apnea:
    A. Can lead to episodes of apnea hundreds of times a night.
    B. Is common among those younger than 30 years of age.
    C. Can be prevented by taking Benadryl for sleeping.
    D. Can be prevented by sleeping in the supine position.

30. A Venturi mask is:
    A. Used for respiratory isolation procedures.
    B. A personal protective piece of equipment.
    C. Used to deliver oxygen according to a prescribed concentration.
    D. Used to deliver oxygen according to a prescribed flow rate.

31. Which of these tuberculosis medications has a side effect of neuropathy?
    A. Isoniazid
    B. Rifampin
    C. Streptomycin
    D. Ethambutol

32. Which of the following is an appropriate nursing diagnosis for a client who has acute respiratory distress syndrome?
    A. Anxiety related to the contagious nature of the acute respiratory distress syndrome
    B. Anxiety related to the need for protective isolation with acute respiratory distress syndrome
    C. Knowledge deficit related to the need for protective isolation
    D. Knowledge deficit related to the need for mechanical ventilation

33. Which disorder is characterized by a paradoxical motion of the chest wall?
    A. Pneumothorax

B. Hemothorax
C. Flail chest
D. Pulmonary embolus

34. Which life-threatening pleural space abnormality is characterized by hyper resonance on the affected side?
    A. Closed pneumothorax
    B. Tension pneumothorax
    C. Flail chest
    D. Pulmonary embolus

35. Which is an appropriate expected outcome for a client taking an opioid for pain?
    A. The client will maintain adequate oxygenation.
    B. The client will be assessed for pain only before the administration of the opioid.
    C. The nurse will assess for pain before administering the opioid.
    D. The nurse will assess for pain before and after administering the opioid.

36. Which nursing diagnosis is appropriate for a client taking an opioid for pain?
    A. At risk for falls
    B. At risk for hypertension
    C. At risk for skin breakdown
    D. At risk for elopement

37. Which of the following risk factors is associated with hospital-acquired pneumonia?
    A. Acute bronchitis
    B. Antacid use
    C. Age over 50
    D. Age over 40

38. Who is at greatest risk for histoplasmosis?
    A. A person who works with asbestos
    B. A person who raises cattle
    C. A frequent visitor to mountain ranges across the nation
    D. A frequent visitor to caves across the nation

39. Which surgical intervention is indicated for well-defined and circumscribed benign and metastatic lung tumors?
    A. Pneumonectomy
    B. Lobectomy
    C. Wedge resection
    D. Decortication

40. Lung volume reduction surgery is indicated for clients who:
    A. Have a forced expiratory volume (FEV_1) of < 40% of the expected.
    B. Have a forced expiratory volume (FEV_1) of < 30% of the expected.

C. Have a forced vital capacity (FVC) of < 70%

D. Have a forced vital capacity (FVC) of < 80%

41. You are teaching your client about the proper use of an incentive spirometer. In which domain of learning are you teaching?
    A. Pulmonary exercises
    B. Pulmonary education
    C. Cognitive
    D. Psychomotor

42. Which teaching strategy is most appropriate when teaching a client about the proper use of an incentive spirometer?
    A. Demonstration
    B. Discussion
    C. Reading material
    D. Role-playing

43. An expected outcome for an educational activity relating to the proper use of an incentive spirometer is:
    A. The nurse will demonstrate the proper use of an incentive spirometer.
    B. The nurse will discuss the importance of an incentive spirometer.
    C. The client will demonstrate the proper use of an incentive spirometer.
    D. The client will discuss the importance of an incentive spirometer.

44. According to the American Association of Critical Care Nurses (AACN), which of the following is one of the eight competencies for progressive care nurses requiring nurses to use evidence-based practices?
    A. Collaboration
    B. Clinical judgment
    C. Systems-thinking
    D. Advocacy

45. Which theorist is credited with General Systems Theory?
    A. Knowles
    B. Maslow
    C. Piaget
    D. Bertalanffy

46. Systems-thinking facilitates:
    A. Self-empowerment.
    B. An organized head-to-toe assessment.
    C. Holistic nursing care.
    D. Priority-setting.

47. Which theorist is credited with the Theory of Transcultural Nursing?
    A. Sister Callista Roy
    B. Madeleine Leininger

C. Dorothea Orem
D. Martha Rogers

48. Madeleine Leininger supports which of the following nursing modes of intervention?
   A. Cultural care restructuring and repatterning
   B. Cultural practices and cultural respect
   C. Self-care agency
   D. Universality

49. Culture impacts which aspects of the teaching/learning process?
   A. Tolerance for low-lighting and low-seating arrangements
   B. The ambient room temperature
   C. The choice of teaching strategies for each domain
   D. Communication and terminology use

50. Which level of stress facilitates learning?
   A. No stress
   B. Low stress
   C. Moderate stress
   D. High stress

51. Which term best describes the progressive care nurse's application of research findings into practice?
   A. Benchmarking practice
   B. Professional decision-making
   C. Critical-thinking practice
   D. Evidence-based practice

52. You give a 10-item multiple choice quiz to a group of clients after teaching a class on cardiac disease and lifestyle choices. Which type of evaluation is this?
   A. Cognitive evaluation
   B. Formative evaluation
   C. Summative evaluation
   D. Interim evaluation

53. A primary purpose of the planning phase of teaching/learning activities is to:
   A. Determine the seating arrangement.
   B. Determine the duration of the session.
   C. Facilitate evaluation.
   D. Determine the teaching strategy.

54. Select the ethical term that is paired with its correct description.
   A. Non-maleficence: "Do not harm," as in the Hippocratic Oath
   B. Beneficence: "Do not harm," as in the Hippocratic Oath

C. Justice: Truthfulness and honesty

D. Fidelity: Fairness and equality

55. Parathyroid secretion is stimulated by falling levels of what?
    A. Sodium
    B. Thyroid hormone
    C. Growth hormone
    D. Plasma calcium

56. A population that is at the greatest risk for hyperparathyroidism is:
    A. Men 25-35 years old.
    B. Men over the age of 60.
    C. Women 30-40 years old.
    D. Women over the age of 60.

57. What is the most serious complication of hypothyroidism?
    A. Severe bone pain
    B. Myxedema coma
    C. Dehydration
    D. Impaired thinking

58. The most serious complication of Addison's disease is:
    A. Adrenal hemorrhage septicemia
    B. Changes in mental status
    C. Bronchospasm
    D. Respiratory alkalosis

59. When palpating the thyroid gland, which assessments can be made?
    A. Consistency and size
    B. Size and mobility
    C. Mobility and consistency
    D. Pain level and mobility

60. Which of the following is NOT one of the 12 cranial nerves?
    A. Olfactory
    B. Optic
    C. Oculomotor
    D. Spinal

61. Normal intracranial pressure is:
    A. 2-10 mmHg.
    B. 5-15 mmHg.

C. 10-15 mmHg.
D. 15-20 mmHg.

62. Cushing's reflex is:
    A. An early sign of brainstem ischemia.
    B. Characterized by tachycardia.
    C. Characterized by hypotension.
    D. A late sign of brainstem ischemia.

63. A widening pulse pressure is a sign of:
    A. Right-sided heart failure.
    B. Left-sided heart failure.
    C. Cheyne-Stokes.
    D. Brainstem herniation.

64. Which type of seizure is paired with its correct description?
    A. Partial seizures: Can be subcategorized as simple partial, complex partial, or secondary generalized seizures.
    B. Generalized seizures: Can be subcategorized as simple partial, complex partial, or secondary generalized seizures.
    C. Non-convulsive seizures: Primarily affect adolescents and young adults.
    D. Generalized tonic-clonic seizures: Previously known as petit mal seizures.

65. Who is at greatest risk for seizures?
    A. A diabetic client with hyperglycemia who is not treated
    B. An actively drinking alcoholic
    C. An adult in a disco with flashing lights
    D. An adult in a loud and noisy restaurant

66. Which type of stroke is paired with its correct description?
    A. Ischemic Stroke: The least frequently occurring type of stroke
    B. Ischemic Stroke: Occurs as the result of an occluded vessel
    C. Hemorrhagic stroke: The most commonly occurring type of stroke
    D. Subarachnoid hemorrhage: Is typically asymptomatic

67. Which type of psychiatric disorder is paired with correct examples of it?
    A. Mood disorders: Dementia and delirium
    B. Gender identity disorders: Anxiety and stress
    C. Personality disorders: Eating disorders and anxiety
    D. Mood disorders: Bi-polar disease and depression

68. The signs and symptoms associated with panic level anxiety include:
    A. Fixed pupils and dizziness.
    B. Chest pain and dizziness.

C. Rambling thoughts and speech.
D. Chest pain and rambling speech.

69. Which psychiatric condition is characterized by the client's feigning of a physical illness?
    A. Munchausen's Syndrome
    B. Munchausen's Syndrome by Proxy
    C. Panic disorder
    D. Depression

70. Suicide is a major life-threatening event among psychiatric clients in hospitals and in the community. Progressive care nurses should:
    A. Not assess those at risk because only a psychiatrist is competent to do so.
    B. Ask the client why he/she is so depressed.
    C. Ask the client, "What are your thoughts now about dying?"
    D. Tell the client that suicide thoughts are a sign of weakness.

71. Which standardized scale is used to assess altered levels of consciousness?
    A. The Glasgow Coma Scale
    B. The Altered Level of Consciousness (LOC) Scale
    C. The Ascending Reticular Activating System (ARAS)
    D. The Descending Reticular Activating System (DRAS)

72. Delirium tremens (DT) are:
    A. Marked with autonomic nervous system hypoactivity.
    B. Characterized by an excess of GABA-A receptor stimulation.
    C. Life-threatening without treatment.
    D. Associated with binge ethanol consumption.

73. Which form of encephalopathy is associated with alcohol abuse?
    A. Hypoxic-ischemic encephalopathy
    B. Hypoxic encephalopathy
    C. Ischemic encephalopathy
    D. Wernicke's encephalopathy

74. Select the type of pain that is paired with its correct description.
    A. Somatic pain: Sharp pain that affects bone, skin, and muscles
    B. Neuropathic pain: The most common type of acute pain
    C. Visceral pain: Tingling, burning, and aching pain
    D. Somatic pain: Cramping, aching, and throbbing pain

75. Your oncology patient is at the end of life and affected with severely significant toxicity relating to his cancer treatment. Which toxicity grade does this patient have as a result of this adverse event?
    A. Toxicity Grade I
    B. Toxicity Grade II

C. Toxicity Grade III
D. Toxicity Grade IV

76. Your patient has just received a kidney transplant. Which nursing diagnosis is most appropriate for her?
    A. Impaired renal function related to an autologous transplantation
    B. At risk for infection related to immunosuppression
    C. Social isolation related to protective isolation
    D. Disuse syndrome related to renal surgery

77. Which client is at greatest risk for multisystem failure?
    A. A client who has just completed radiation therapy and has an indwelling catheter
    B. A client who has just completed radiation therapy and has a central line
    C. A client who has just completed chemotherapy and has an indwelling catheter
    D. A client who has just completed chemotherapy through a central line

78. The primary cause of nosocomial vancomycin-resistant enterococcus (VRE) is:
    A. Overuse of cephalosporin drugs.
    B. Use of central venous lines.
    C. Use of indwelling urinary catheters
    D. Presence of methicillin-resistant staphylococcus aureus superbug.

79. Which type of shock occurs when excessive nitric oxide leads to massive vasodilation?
    A. Septic shock
    B. Anaphylactic shock
    C. Hypovolemic shock
    D. Systemic inflammatory response

80. Which client is at greatest risk for noninfectious systemic inflammatory response syndrome (SIRS)?
    A. A client with a central venous line
    B. A client with an indwelling urinary catheter
    C. A client with a 3rd-degree burn
    D. A client with an anterior wall myocardial infarction

81. While teaching your patient about proper diet, you notice that he has a fruity breath odor. Which disorder would you most likely suspect?
    A. Failure to thrive
    B. Metabolic syndrome
    C. Malabsorption
    D. Ketoacidosis

82. A complication of diabetic ketoacidosis is:
   A. Hyperkalemia.
   B. Hypokalemia.
   C. Hypercalcemia.
   D. Hypocalcemia.

83. Your client has atrial fibrillation and is being successfully treated with Coumadin. Which expected outcome is most appropriate for her?
   A. The client will be free of aplastic anemia
   B. The client will verbalize a knowledge of the INR test
   C. Knowledge deficit related to atrial fibrillation
   D. Knowledge deficit related to Coumadin

84. Your client had a coronary artery bypass grafting (CABG) four days ago and is receiving heparin. Which nursing diagnosis is most appropriate for him?
   A. At risk for thrombocytopenia
   B. At risk for anaphylactic shock
   C. At risk for aplastic anemia
   D. At risk for atrial fibrillation

85. Cardiac tamponade is a risk factor for which disorder?
   A. Impaired Ascending Reticular Activating System (ARAS)
   B. Impaired Descending Reticular Activating System (DRAS)
   C. Korsakoff's syndrome
   D. Systemic inflammatory response syndrome (SIRS)

86. Which type of leukemia is associated with a white blood cell count of 20,000-100,000/mm^3?
   A. Chronic myelogenous leukemia
   B. Chronic lymphoblastic leukemia
   C. Acute myelogenous leukemia
   D. Acute lymphoblastic leukemia

87. Your postoperative appendectomy client has absent bowel signs in all four quadrants. Which disorder would you most likely suspect?
   A. A bowel obstruction
   B. Infection
   C. A paralytic ileus
   D. A paralytic ileum

88. Your diabetic client is experiencing severe nausea and vomiting. Which disorder would you most likely suspect?
   A. Irritable bowel syndrome
   B. Gastroesophageal reflux
   C. Dumping syndrome
   D. Gastroparesis

89. Irritable bowel syndrome is treated with:
    A. Psychotherapy.
    B. Antacids.
    C. Statin drugs.
    D. Anticholinergic drugs.

90. Upper gastrointestinal hemorrhage is associated with:
    A. Alcoholic esophageal varices.
    B. Crohn's disease.
    C. Cushing's syndrome.
    D. Colon strictures.

91. Your client is experiencing encephalopathy, bleeding, jaundice, drowsiness, and a swollen abdomen. Which disorder would you most likely suspect?
    A. End-stage renal disease
    B. Hepatic failure
    C. Common bile duct obstruction
    D. Bowel obstruction

92. Chronic pancreatitis can present with which symptoms?
    A. Steatorrhea and lower abdominal pain
    B. Steatorrhea and weight gain
    C. Weight loss and steatorrhea
    D. Lower abdominal pain and indigestion

93. The initial treatment of acute pancreatitis includes:
    A. The complete cessation of eating and drinking.
    B. Intravenous diuretics.
    C. Intravenous cholinergics.
    D. A dietary protein and sodium restriction.

94. A complication of renal failure is:
    A. Muscular spasticity.
    B. Encephalopathy.
    C. Shortness of breath.
    D. Malabsorption.

95. Which disorder does your type 2 diabetic patient most likely have when her blood glucose levels are extremely high without the presence of ketones?
    A. Ketotic hyperglycemic hyperosmolar coma
    B. Diabetic hypoglycemic hyperosmolar syndrome
    C. Diabetic hyperglycemic hyperosmolar syndrome
    D. Ketotic hyperglycemic hypomolar coma

96. Which type of anemia is treated with vitamin B12?
   A. Aplastic anemia
   B. Iron deficiency anemia
   C. Pernicious anemia
   D. Chronic anemia

97. Which statement about failure to thrive is accurate?
   A. Failure to thrive can occur when a patient has cystic fibrosis.
   B. Failure to thrive has only psychosocial risk factors.
   C. Failure to thrive is most common among the elderly.
   D. Failure to thrive can occur when a patient has transient syncope.

98. Transient ischemic attacks:
   A. Lead to only minor permanent neurological damage.
   B. Do not lead to permanent neurological damage.
   C. Lead to temporary aphasia and hemiparesis when posterior circulation is impaired.
   D. Lead to temporary hemiparesis and dysphagia when anterior circulation is impaired.

99. Transient ischemic attacks are treated with:
   A. Acute care hospitalization for at least four days for the treatment of hypertension.
   B. Supplemental oxygen and antiplatelet medications.
   C. Acute care hospitalization for at least five days for stabilization.
   D. Platelets and supplemental oxygen therapy.

100.   The FAST pneumonic for the signs and symptoms of stroke includes:
   A. F (flaccidity), A (atony), S (sluggish pupils), and T (treatment)
   B. F (focal seizure), A (arm weakness), S (speech changes), and T (treatment)
   C. F (facial weakness), A (arm weakness), S (syncope), and T (time)
   D. F (facial weakness), A (arm weakness), S (speech changes), and T (time is of the essence)

Test Your Knowledge—Answers

1. B	23. C	45. D	67. D
2. A	24. A	46. C	68. B
3. D	25. A	47. B	69. A
4. D	26. C	48. A	70. C
5. B	27. D	49. D	71. A
6. C	28. B	50. C	72. C
7. A	29. A	51. D	73. D
8. C	30. C	52. C	74. A
9. B	31. A	53. C	75. C
10. D	32. D	54. A	76. B
11. A	33. C	55. D	77. D
12. C	34. B	56. D	78. A
13. C	35. A	57. B	79. A
14. B	36. A	58. A	80. C
15. A	37. B	59. A	81. D
16. A	38. D	60. D	82. B
17. A	39. C	61. B	83. B
18. C	40. B	62. D	84. A
19. D	41. D	63. D	85. D
20. D	42. A	64. A	86. B
21. C	43. C	65. C	87. C
22. A	44. B	66. B	88. D

89. A	92. C	95. C	98. B
90. A	93. A	96. C	99. B
91. B	94. C	97. A	100. D

Exclusive Trivium Test Tips

Here at Trivium Test Prep, we strive to offer you the exemplary test tools that help you pass your exam the first time. This book includes an overview of important concepts, example questions throughout the text, and practice test questions. But we know that learning how to successfully take a test can be just as important as learning the content being tested. In addition to excelling on the PCCN, we want to give you the solutions you need to be successful every time you take a test. Our study strategies, preparation pointers, and test tips will help you succeed as you take the PCCN and any test in the future!

Study Strategies

1. Spread out your studying. By taking the time to study a little bit every day, you strengthen your understanding of the testing material, so it's easier to recall that information on the day of the test. Our study guides make this easy by breaking up the concepts into sections with example practice questions, so you can test your knowledge as you read.

2. Create a study calendar. The sections of our book make it easy to review and practice with example questions on a schedule. Decide to read a specific number of pages or complete a number of practice questions every day. Breaking up all of the information in this way can make studying less overwhelming and more manageable.

3. Set measurable goals and motivational rewards. Follow your study calendar and reward yourself for completing reading, example questions, and practice problems and tests. You could take yourself out after a productive week of studying or watch a favorite show after reading a chapter. Treating yourself to rewards is a great way to stay motivated.

4. Use your current knowledge to understand new, unfamiliar concepts. When you learn something new, think about how it relates to something you know really well. Making connections between new ideas and your existing understanding can simplify the learning process and make the new information easier to remember.

5. Make learning interesting! If one aspect of a topic is interesting to you, it can make an entire concept easier to remember. Stay engaged and think about how concepts covered on the exam can affect the things you're interested in. The sidebars throughout the text offer additional information that could make ideas easier to recall.

6. Find a study environment that works for you. For some people, absolute silence in a library results in the most effective study session, while others need the background noise of a coffee shop to fuel productive studying. There are many websites that generate white noise and recreate the sounds of different environments for studying. Figure out what distracts you and what engages you and plan accordingly.

7. Take practice tests in an environment that reflects the exam setting. While it's important to be as comfortable as possible when you study, practicing taking the test exactly as you'll take it on test day will make you more prepared for the actual exam. If your test starts on a Saturday morning, take your practice test on a Saturday morning. If you have access, try to find an empty classroom that has desks like the desks at testing center. The more closely you can mimic the testing center, the more prepared you'll feel on test day.

8. Study hard for the test in the days before the exam, but take it easy the night before and do something relaxing rather than studying and cramming. This will help decrease anxiety, allow you to get a better night's sleep, and be more mentally fresh during the big exam. Watch a light-hearted movie, read a favorite book, or take a walk, for example.

Preparation Pointers

1. Preparation is key! Don't wait until the day of your exam to gather your pencils, calculator, identification materials, or admission tickets. Check the requirements of the exam as soon as possible. Some tests require materials that may take more time to obtain, such as a passport-style photo, so be sure that you have plenty of time to collect everything. The night before the exam, lay out everything you'll need, so it's all ready to go on test day! We recommend at least two forms of ID, your admission ticket or confirmation, pencils, a high protein, compact snack, bottled water, and any necessary medications. Some testing centers will require you to put all of your supplies in a clear plastic bag. If you're prepared, you will be less stressed the morning of, and less likely to forget anything important.

2. If you're taking a pencil-and-paper exam, test your erasers on paper. Some erasers leave big, dark stains on paper instead of rubbing out pencil marks. Make sure your erasers work for you and the pencils you plan to use.

3. Make sure you give yourself your usual amount of sleep, preferably at least 7 – 8 hours. You may find you need even more sleep. Pay attention to how much you sleep in the days before the exam, and how many hours it takes for you to feel refreshed. This will allow you to be as sharp as possible during the test and make fewer simple mistakes.

4. Make sure to make transportation arrangements ahead of time, and have a backup plan in case your ride falls through. You don't want to be stressing about how you're going to get to the testing center the morning of the exam.

5. Many testing locations keep their air conditioners on high. You want to remember to bring a sweater or jacket in case the test center is too cold, as you never know how hot or cold the testing location could be. Remember, while you can always adjust for heat by removing layers, if you're cold, you're cold.

Test Tips

1. Go with your gut when choosing an answer. Statistically, the answer that comes to mind first is often the right one. This is assuming you studied the material, of course, which we hope you have done if you've read through one of our books!

2. For true or false questions: if you genuinely don't know the answer, mark it true. In most tests, there are typically more true answers than false answers.

3. For multiple-choice questions, read ALL the answer choices before marking an answer, even if you think you know the answer when you come across it. You may find your original "right" answer isn't necessarily the best option.

4. Look for key words: in multiple choice exams, particularly those that require you to read through a text, the questions typically contain key words. These key words can help the test taker choose the correct answer or confuse you if you don't recognize them. Common keywords are: *most*, *during*, *after*, *initially*, and *first*. Be sure you identify them before you read the available answers. Identifying the key words makes a huge difference in your chances of passing the test.

5. Narrow answers down by using the process of elimination: after you understand the question, read each answer. If you don't know the answer right away, use the process of elimination to narrow down the answer choices. It is easy to identify at least one answer that isn't correct. Continue to narrow down the choices before choosing the answer you believe best fits the question. By following this process, you increase your chances of selecting the correct answer.

6. Don't worry if others finish before or after you. Go at your own pace, and focus on the test in front of you.

7. Relax. With our help, we know you'll be ready to conquer the PCCN. You've studied and worked hard!

Keep in mind that every individual takes tests differently, so strategies that might work for you may not work for someone else. You know yourself best and are the best person to determine which of these tips and strategies will benefit your studying and test taking. Best of luck as you study, test, and work toward your future!

PCCN Essential Test Tips Video
from Trivium Test Prep!

Dear Customer,

Thank you for purchasing from Trivium Test Prep! We're honored to help you prepare for your PCCN exam.

To show our appreciation, we're offering a **FREE** *PCCN Essential Test Tips* **Video by Trivium Test Prep**. Our Video includes 35 test preparation strategies that will make you successful on the PCCN. All we ask is that you email us your feedback and describe your experience with our product. Amazing, awful, or just so-so: we want to hear what you have to say!

To receive your **FREE** *PCCN Essential Test Tips* **Video**, please email us at 5star@triviumtestprep.com. Include "Free 5 Star" in the subject line and the following information in your email:

1. The title of the product you purchased.
2. Your rating from 1 – 5 (with 5 being the best).
3. Your feedback about the product, including how our materials helped you meet your goals and ways in which we can improve our products.
4. Your full name and shipping address so we can send your FREE *PCCN Essential Test Tips* Video.

If you have any questions or concerns please feel free to contact us directly at 5star@triviumtestprep.com.

Thank you!

CPSIA information can be obtained
at www.ICGtesting.com
Printed in the USA
BVHW051027080421
604340BV00008B/544